Sugar Happy
For Happy Blood Sugars

Diabetes Health Guide

By
Nadia Al-Samarrie
Diabetes Advocate

King's Publishing Inc.

Woodacre, California, USA

Copyright© Nadia Al-Samarrie, 2018, 2019, 2020

ISBN: 978-1-7323477-4-8

DISCLAIMER

The information in this book is not intended nor implied to be a substitute for professional medical advice, diagnosis or treatment. All content in this book is for general purposes only. Never disregard professional medical advice or delay seeking medical treatment because of something you have read in this book.

Neither the author nor the publisher assumes any responsibility for errors, omissions, or contrary interpretations of the subject matter herein. Any perceived slight of any individual or organization is purely unintentional.

Brand and product names are trademarks or registered trademarks of their respective owners.

Editing: Patrick Totty

DEDICATION

Without my mother

Without my brother

Without my aunt

Without my grandmothers

Before I knew I would lose them to diabetes, I was their advocate.

I hope this book will inspire you to do your personal best in delaying or preventing diabetes complications.

CONTENTS

INTRODUCTION
WHY DIABETES IS OVERWHELMING

Over the past twenty-eight years, I have learned that no matter how educated you are, being diabetes literate makes a difference. Having spent time in the company of friends and family who have diabetes, I have been able to observe first-hand how important it is to understand how to live with diabetes. Diabetes is not something you can cure, but it should not stop you from living a long and happy life.

My former husband was diagnosed with type 1 diabetes at the age of 17. He knows a lot about his disease. He understands how food affects him, how much insulin he needs to take, what type of insulin to take, and when to take it. As a result, he has successfully lived with diabetes for more than forty years, and in his early sixties, leads an active and healthy life.

Sugar Happy

In contrast to my former husband are my grandmother, my mother, my brother, and my aunt, Grace. They all had type 2 diabetes, and despite being knowledgeable about many things in life, they did not learn to manage their diabetes. For years they struggled unsuccessfully to maintain their health with little true understanding of what they needed to do, and eventually, they all passed away from complications of the disease.

By the time she was in her fifties, my mother had thyroid issues, high cholesterol, and high blood pressure. She was used to taking medications. So, what was adding diabetes to her cluster of diseases? At the time, it seemed as if all she had to do was take another pill, and she would be fine. This lack of understanding of diabetes and the cumulative effect that it could have on overall health led to her demise. She rated each day as being either good or bad without thinking of the long-term consequences of the numerous "bad" days. Her attitude was always that tomorrow was going to be a different day. In most cases, it was not.

My brother, Jamal, was diagnosed with type 2 diabetes at the age of 40. I didn't know he had diabetes until he came to visit us in the U.S. for his 50th birthday. As a young kid, Jamal was a super athlete. In high school, he was a charmer; the girls called him Don Juan. His grades in class were either F's or A's, never in between. He could sit down, listen to a song on the radio, and then play it on our piano without ever having taken a piano lesson. He also had a photographic memory. My siblings and I agreed hands down that he could have been a rocket scientist if he had wanted to. At the time of his diagnosis, Jamal lived in Australia, where he had access to excellent medical care. Yet when I saw him on his last visit to the U.S., he looked gaunt, walked slowly, and had not slept through the night in years.

I showed Jamal how to manage his blood sugars and explained that if he was going to the bathroom three times throughout the evening, it could be because of high blood sugars. He got a glucose meter to test this theory. He learned about carbohydrate counting, and we found him a physician who put him on insulin. When he left the U.S. a month later, he had a skip in his walk. In fact, he called me from the airport to thank me for helping him figure out what he needed to do. Yet without continued support, Jamal passed away within five years.

Aunt Grace, a type 2 diabetic, was another brilliant person. She was at my birth in Baghdad, and we share the same birthday. She had two master's degrees from Berkeley and was exceptionally well-read, yet she too seemed unable to grasp the importance of controlling her blood sugar levels. When I saw her at my mother's memorial, she did not look well. I asked her to check her blood sugar reading. She took it, and to our surprise, her blood sugar was 600 milligrams per deciliter. The normal range before a meal is 70 to 130 milligrams per deciliter, but despite having insulin available, Aunt Grace regularly ran her blood sugars high. When she passed away soon after a stroke, a common complication of diabetes, I was shocked but not surprised.

Sugar Happy

My grandmother in Baghdad also had type 2 diabetes. Her self-imposed therapy was using Sweet 'n Low in her tea. She ate chocolates, privately smoked cigarettes, had excess weight, and did not understand how food affected her blood sugar because no one taught her. This was back in the late '70s. There was not much in diabetes education back then nor a community to learn from.

What do all these people have in common? They did not understand their diabetes and how it affected them. Food, stress, grief, illness, medication, medical devices, managing blood sugars, sleep, planning travel, holiday, and family parties, are many variables that can impact your blood sugar.

My diabetes family has been a significant influence in my life. So many people whom I've loved never became diabetes literate, regardless of their educational background. They never learned how different foods, exercise, or checking their blood sugars affected them. They assumed at their diagnosis that since their physician had given them a prescription, that the pill would take care of everything. They resumed their lives with type 2 diabetes but with no lifestyle changes.

I learned so much from my former husband, who had already been living with type 1 for 11 years when I first met him. He made managing his diabetes look easy. You eat, you take insulin, you check your blood sugar, and you exercise. That supposed ease frustrated my mother to no avail. She struggled with her diabetes because, again, she did not learn what she needed to know. At the end of her life, she finally got it. However, unfortunately, it was too late.

Why Diabetes Is Overwhelming

After getting married in the eighties and working corporate jobs, both my husband and I decided we were not corporate people. We opened a diabetes mail order store in San Francisco with the idea of moving to the country and raising a family someday. The business grew quickly. Six months into it, we found ourselves producing and hosting a diabetes radio show in which specialists in diabetes care participated. Listeners could call in and ask a question, and the experts shared their knowledge. Shortly after we started the radio show, we were asked if we could transcribe the shows. In less than two years, we had a mail-order business, a radio show, and a magazine.

For the next six years, I spoke with people with type 1 and type 2 diabetes, parents of children with diabetes, and pregnant women who were diagnosed with gestational diabetes. I learned so much during that time. Added to that, I was on my own emotional roller coaster with my mother, dealing with her diabetes complications. The realization that there was little I could do to help her if she was not willing to be diabetes literate, served to inspire me to continue in my efforts to educate others. The mental games she played with herself exhausted me but have served as my greatest inspiration.

My family, friends, former husband, Sugar Happy Diabetes Supplies customers, DiabetesHealth.Com subscribers, podcast guests, video interviews, and the inquiries that pour in from my *AskNadia* column are my collective inspiration for this book. Their shared success and concerns can now be your inspiration in creating a real change in your diabetes self-management. Adversely, their stories, like my mother, grandmother, aunt, and brother, can also be a cautionary tale as to the pitfalls of a lack of diabetes literacy.

This book, *Sugar Happy,* will also help family members, parents, grandparents, and employers to understand the complexity of living with diabetes. My advice to you, as a support provider, is to not oversimplify what you think the person is feeling nor tell them what they should or should not do. Instead, offer to be a support system with their permission. Do not police the person living with diabetes. They are already doing it to themselves regardless of what you may perceive. Unless you are living with a metabolic disorder, you likely have no idea how the disease can personally impact a person living with diabetes.

This book will also illuminate living with a pre-diabetes diagnosis, as it lays out the psychological, biological, and treatment for diabetes. I believe if people with a pre-diabetes diagnosis really understood how complex the disease is, more effort would be put in preventing a diagnosis of diabetes. There is no cure for type 2 diabetes. The only way to delay or prevent a diagnosis is to make the lifestyle changes required to achieve better health.

Your Personal Take Away Notes To Remember

CHAPTER 1

UNDERSTANDING DIABETES

Diabetes in your family tree does not guarantee a diagnosis. However, if you have an unhealthy lifestyle or a genetic predisposition to it, a diagnosis is likely.

My great-grandmother, both my grandmothers, mother, brother, and aunt all had diabetes. There was a time in their lives during their pre-diabetes phase when their glucose levels were higher than average, allowing them to adjust their lifestyles. They could have possibly delayed or prevented a diabetes diagnosis.

Growing up, I thought medication was all that was needed to manage diabetes. Later as I matured, I learned a lot more about my family's predisposition to diabetes and what was really needed to successfully manage it. Consequently, when I take my annual glucose test and A1c test, if my blood glucose results are a bit elevated from the previous year or near the pre-diabetes range, I adjust my diet and start exercising more to delay or prevent my diagnosis. After making dietary changes, my next glucose test always reads at a lower A1c, showing me that my little lifestyle changes helped in lowering my blood sugar level.

What is Diabetes?

Diabetes is a condition in which your pancreas does not make enough insulin, or your body does not sufficiently use the insulin manufactured. When you eat certain food and drinks, they turn into sugar in your bloodstream. You cannot have high levels of sugar floating in your blood without it affecting your overall health. Sugar binds to proteins, making your arteries look like turkey jerky. This condition can impede blood flow and be dangerous to your health.

So, the pancreas releases insulin into your bloodstream, thereby converting the glucose from your bloodstream into energy in your cells. With the help of insulin, your cells will be able to either use the energy from sugar or store it. With the right amount of insulin, your blood sugar will stabilize, and your cells will be fed. But if you have diabetes, there is a disruption in this process. Why? You could be insulin-resistant (i.e., your blood cells are unable to use your insulin effectively, which can lead to high blood sugar), or you could be not producing enough insulin, and this is what diabetes is all about. It is important to note that some people have other conditions that may contribute to their diabetes diagnosis, such as sickle cell disease, thyroid dysfunction, being pregnant, or using medications that can increase blood sugar, such as steroids or some cholesterol medications. All of these increase the risk of a diabetes diagnosis.

You Are Not Alone

The National Institute of Diabetes and Digestive and Kidney Diseases estimated that 84.1 million people in the United States have pre-diabetes, which is a staggering 25.5% of the U.S. population for adults who are 18 or over.

If you have been diagnosed with diabetes, then you are one of the 23.1 million people who are aware of their diagnosis. Another 7.2 million people have diabetes and don't know it, making them susceptible to diabetes complications.

The American Diabetes Association reports 1.5 million people are living with type 1 diabetes in the U.S.

Diabetes Symptoms Before Diagnosis

If you have been diagnosed with diabetes, you may have experienced:

- blurry vision
- lethargy
- unquenchable thirst
- visiting the restroom frequently
- fluctuations in your weight
- sores that took a long time to heal

Sugar Happy

- tingling or pain in your hands and feet
- a recommendation by your dentist to get a blood glucose test after looking at your swollen, red gums

These are some of the common symptoms of diabetes, but this list is not exhaustive. You may have one, some, all, or even none of these symptoms. If you do experience them, the symptoms could come on quickly or slowly. There is no set standard, as everyone is different. If you are not aware of any symptom, then it is helpful to be regularly checked for diabetes if you have any of these risk factors:

Seasonal Diagnosis

Interestingly, there is a seasonal diagnosis for certain types of diabetes. The World Health Organization's Diabetes Mondiale (DiaMond) Project conducted a 10-year study with 53 countries to determine the worldwide incidence of type 1 diabetes among children ages 14 and under. An additional study used the results of this research to determine if there was a seasonal pattern in the diagnosis of type 1 diabetes in these children. This study found that 40% (42 of the 105 centers) reported a higher instance of type 1 diabetes for this age group during the summer months in Southern Sweden. However, the incidence of type 2 diabetes diagnoses seemed immune to seasonal changes.

Different Types of Diabetes

Pre-diabetes

Pre-diabetes is when your glucose level is high but not high enough to be diagnosed with diabetes. The current A1c range for a pre-diabetes diagnosis is 5.7%–6.4%. If you have pre-diabetes, you are in the early stages of your insulin not working efficiently to convert the glucose from your blood into your cells for energy. However, it is not too late to make a change.

This is a significant time for your health, and you may be able to avoid a possible diabetes diagnosis by making lifestyle changes, such as watching what you eat, exercising regularly, and visiting your healthcare provider to stay on top of your health. (See chapter 2 for more on lifestyle changes.) This may be easier said than done because the diagnosis typically comes when we are already entrenched in unhealthy habits. You have to make a conscious decision about your health once your healthcare provider tells you that you have been diagnosed with pre-diabetes.

Type 1 Diabetes

Formerly called *juvenile diabetes*. This form of diabetes was once defined as insulin-dependent diabetes for children under the age of 18. Today, type 1 diabetes can be diagnosed at any age, changing the medical diagnosis term from *juvenile diabetes* to *type 1 diabetes, insulin-dependent diabetes,* or *insulin-dependent diabetes mellitus.*

Sugar Happy

Type 1 diabetes is classified as an auto-immune disease where the beta cells in the pancreas no longer function to create insulin, thus creating a void in regulating the glucose levels in your body. Since insulin converts food into energy, your body needs this hormone to work correctly.

In the U.S., there are 1.5 million adults and children with type 1 diabetes. The cure for type 1 diabetes has been promised for almost six decades now. Once hopeful families, with children with diabetes have lost faith in a cure from conventional research organizations and nonprofits. As a result, many type 1 non-profits have formed to focus more aggressively on finding the cure. Parents of children with type 1 diabetes lead the way in starting these organizations by sitting on the boards and fundraising.

Research is still unable to ascertain why the pancreas stops making insulin. There are many theories but nothing conclusive. Experts continue to seek an explanation as to why the autoimmune systems attack the beta cells, the insulin-producing hormones. For families with children with diabetes and adults with type 1 diabetes, the focus is on daily management to avoid complications with the continued long-term hope for a cure.

Type 1.5 Diabetes

Type 1.5 diabetes, also known as Latent Autoimmune Diabetes in Adults (LADA), is an autoimmune disease that falls between type 1 and type 2 diabetes because it has characteristics of both.

According to an article in The Beacon News, approximately 10 percent of patients with type 1.5 are misdiagnosed with type 2. If you're over 35 when you develop diabetes, and especially if you have excess weight or classified as obese, your healthcare provider may assume that you have type 2 diabetes.

Therefore, if you don't quite fit the profile of someone with type 2 diabetes, if diabetes pills don't seem to be working well, or if you show some of the characteristics of type 1, maybe you have LADA. People with LADA have islet antibodies in their blood, and as in type 1 diabetes, their immune system is attacking beta cells. However, this is happening at a much slower rate and initially, they don't need insulin. One may consider that LADA is type 1 diabetes that progresses slowly.

One study in Diabetes Care states you probably have LADA (rather than type 2 diabetes) if two or more of the following fit:

- You were under age 50 when you were diagnosed with diabetes.
- You had "acute" symptoms at diagnosis, that is, symptoms typical of type 1 diabetes.
- Your BMI is less than 25.
- You have a personal history of autoimmune disease (such as thyroid disease, celiac sprue, Addison's disease, or others).
- You have a family history of autoimmune disease.

Sugar Happy

The symptoms of type 1.5 are the same as the more well-known types of diabetes. They include increased thirst, increased urination, weight loss, and blurred vision.

Type 2 Diabetes

Historically, type 2 diabetes was found in mature adults over 40 who have a family history of diabetes, a sedentary lifestyle, and excess weight. Today, these statistics have changed, as obesity has risen in the youth population. According to the 2017 National Diabetes Statistics Report, it was estimated that 5,300 children ages 10–19 were diagnosed with type 2 diabetes from 2011 to 2012.

Type 2 diabetes can typically be managed with diet and exercise, but type 2 medications or insulin may also be required.

Overcoming the Shock of Being Diagnosed with Diabetes

Pre-diabetes

People diagnosed with pre-diabetes and who are concerned about an eventual diabetes diagnosis can make immediate lifestyle changes to help delay or prevent diabetes.

I have friends and family members who understand pre-diabetes, but, to my amazement, few make the lifestyle changes necessary, such as increasing their physical activity or watching what they eat.

Type 1 Children

If you are a parent and your child has been diagnosed with type 1 diabetes, your first reaction may be fear. When I had a diabetes supply store in San Francisco, I spoke to many parents with newly diagnosed children. Their biggest fear was having their child fall into a coma from low blood sugar (a hypoglycemic event) and die.

Imagine taking your 5-year-old, newly diagnosed child to kindergarten, saying goodbye for the day, and leaving them at school, fearing they may experience low blood sugar, but no one knows how to help them. How's that going to work out? High blood sugar (hyperglycemia) is not good either, but the parent's fear is usually about low blood sugar and having people around who know how to treat it or will call an ambulance in time. My children were in an elementary school where their teacher took a diabetes education class in case she needed to help her student. I was impressed by her. It is not common for teachers to take diabetes educational classes to help one student. But, Amy Valens has always been a stand out in her field.

The second comment parents usually made to me was, "I wish I had it and not my child." As parents, we suffer when we feel our children are hurt. When it comes to a chronic medical condition, there is so much that is out of our control.

For the parents who came into my medical supply store, online diabetes communities did not exist. I assisted them in starting a network with one another as moral support. Over time, when they came back into the store, they thanked me because it helped them to know that another parent shared their fears regarding their child's safety daily, 24/7.

Sugar Happy

Type 1 Adults

Newly diagnosed adults who came into Sugar Happy Diabetes Supplies had a different response to their diagnosis. Most of the symptoms they had experienced came to an end when they began treatment, offering relief and an explanation. At the same time, surrendering to a new condition required patience and overcoming their fear of a possible fatal hypoglycemic event.

Though many of my customers blamed themselves for lifestyle choices, some were slim, ate organically, did not drink alcohol or coffee, and were vegetarians. They told me they felt like God was punishing them.

Adults who were diagnosed with type 1 diabetes in their 50s told me it took a while to get used to diabetes self-management. They, of course, like the parents of children with type 1 diabetes, were concerned about all the possible complications and hypoglycemia, driving them to use all the available medical technology to manage their blood sugars.

Type 2 Diabetes

In my personal and professional experience, people who are diagnosed with type 2 diabetes either embrace it and create positive lifestyle changes or remain in a state of denial. I have two friends with husbands who were diagnosed with type 2 diabetes, and they each made immediate lifestyle changes after their diagnosis. They changed their diet to eating less carbohydrates and started exercising daily, even if it was just a walk after a meal. My type 2 family members, on the other hand, took their medication but did not change their diet or exercise regularly. Over time, my family's inability to make these simple changes shortened their lifespans.

My conversations with people living successfully with type 2 diabetes were motivated by their fears of going blind, possible amputations, suffering diabetes complications, and/or their quality of life, possibly becoming limited.

For people with type 1 and type 2, a diabetes diagnosis can affect self- esteem, making them feel helpless. Some people have told me they feel like damaged goods. I had one customer tell me that when she was younger, a man who had diabetes wanted to marry her. She refused his proposal because he had diabetes. Ironically, she was in my store buying diabetes supplies for the man she chose to marry who did not have diabetes at the time of their wedding.

In our discussion, I mentioned that my husband had type 1 diabetes. She looked at me wide-eyed, pushed her head back with surprise, and said: "You mean you knew he had diabetes, and you still married him?" You can imagine where that conversation went next — nowhere. But my talk with her helped me to understand the fears and vulnerability that people with diabetes have in addition to any physical complications that may transpire.

How Does Your Family Manage Health Issues?

My mother modeled her diabetes care after her mother. Grandmother Helen was in her mid-seventies and in a nursing home.

Sugar Happy

Every time I went to visit her, she was happy and surprised at my sudden arrival. She quickly started stuffing candy wrappers underneath her mattress before my mother made it into her room. She passed away at the nursing home. I am not sure what they wrote as the cause of her death, but my experience tells me her blood sugars were most likely consistently high for a prolonged period. This was back in the early '70s when glucose testing was not what it is today and not frequently checked.

One friend called me a while back because her grandmother was in the hospital. She asked if her grandmother's blood sugar of 600 was OK. She said the medical staff said they like to keep the blood sugars of their elderly patients a bit high. I told her if it were my family member, I would ask them to treat her, bringing down her blood sugar. I have heard that some healthcare professionals like to keep the blood sugar levels of the elderly a bit higher, but 600? A diabetes specialist on staff, such as a physician or a certified diabetes educator, would think differently than non-specialists. This is not to say that all medical staff at a healthcare facility won't bring down a patient's high blood sugar without a diabetes specialist or an educator there to guide them, but having that specialist on hand can be helpful.

Sometimes the patient and the healthcare provider worry more about lowering high blood sugar than raising low blood sugar. And for the patient, lowering high blood sugar can be scary, even causing fear of death. For some healthcare professionals and facilities, the worry is more about the liability of being sued for low blood sugar, should the patient get too low. This is a real concern for some physicians causing a delay in putting their patients on insulin.

As a diabetes patient advocate, I can tell you, diabetes or not; everyone needs an advocate when they go to a medical facility such as a hospital or a living care facility. Recently, I visited a family member who was in the emergency room. It was cold, and she needed a blanket. The nurse ignored her request for one. I had to walk out into the hall and flag someone down to get a blanket. The attending nurse did not take care of her, not because the room was full, or he was busy, but because he felt his patient's request was not necessary. Even though it is his job to make the patient, he is tending, comfortable.

It was only after overhearing a conversation that I had with a physician, about whom I had written an article, that the attending nurse suddenly took great interest in us. He started to check in to ensure that we were comfortable and that all was going well. In fact, when the time came for us to leave, he even walked us out and opened the exit door for us.

When you are hospitalized or have to be cared for in a long-term facility, an informed advocate goes a long way toward ensuring that you get the best care possible.

What Is Modeled for You

One day, as we lay in her hospital bed watching TV, I asked my mother, who was legally blind from her diabetes, how she felt after her vascular surgery. Her response reflected how she managed her diabetes over the years. She said, "If I knew what I know now, I would have managed my diabetes differently. I saw how my mother took care of her diabetes and she was fine and lived into her 70s. I thought the same thing would happen to me."

I, on the other hand, have seen enough family members suffer from diabetes complications. In a backhanded way, I can say my family modeled what *not* to do when it comes to health and diabetes self-management.

Your Personal Take Away Notes To Remember

CHAPTER 2
FEARING DIABETES

Having diabetes can feel overwhelming and create lots of fears. After diagnosis, people start remembering all the horrible things they

have heard or seen, like going blind, getting limbs amputated, going into a coma, decreasing their quality of life, or imminent doom.

Let's address death first. It gives me great comfort to know that we all have the same ending on Earth; we merely take different roads. Death is imminent for us all, so there is no need to fear it. It is going to happen, willingly or unwillingly. Don't fear dying.

Diabetes complications, on the other hand, is something you need to pay attention to. It can shorten or extend your life, in either case with or without pain. You are the only person who has full control over your health. Don't take it for granted. Not everyone lives through being a teenager, twenty-something, or middle age. If you are reading my book, I applaud you. You made it this far. Don't screw it up now by not making the changes needed to avoid or delay diabetes complications.

The reality is diabetes today is more manageable than ever. The biggest hurdle is making the necessary changes. You need to be willing to create change in your life for the best possible outcome. Change requires that you let go of old habits and replace them with new habits. These new habits require new thoughts because the brain is the engine that runs the body.

Diabetes self-management requires education, implementation, a healthcare team, and letting go of blame or shame. It does not matter which type of diabetes you have; once you have the diagnosis, it becomes the beginning of a new life.

Before I started my diabetes supply medical business in San Francisco, I hated my job as a stockbroker. I loved stocks and investing, but the work environment was toxic. The office manager was having an affair with his secretary, which was challenging to witness as I had met his wife and kids at an office picnic. The woman who sat next to me at the office had had a heart attack. The company hired sleazy boiler room guys from an investment company that was closed down and being investigated.

Two associate brokers used to call my extension after hours, as I worked late to build my business. They put our conversation on speaker, pretending to be big investors so they could ridicule and mock me. I called them out on it and hung up, just letting it roll off my back. There was one man in particular, who always called me "honey." Every encounter I had with him, I reminded him that my name was Nadia. He refused to call me by my first name.

One stockbroker was deemed a role model in our sales meetings; his success was considered something to aspire to. When the Security Exchange Commission came and handcuffed him at the office, the office manager lowered his head and shook it, as if he and upper management had no idea what was going on.

When friends and family asked me what it was like to be a stockbroker, I told them to watch the movie *Wall Street*. I felt such relief being able to share my work environment on a large theater screen.

I hated my job and desperately needed to create change. I knew if I extended my employment, it was just a matter of time before I had a health crisis. The conflict? I had done so much to get there. As a bicultural person with an ethnic name, finding employment in a white male dominant work environment was not easy. The Bachelor of Science, a business college degree, and working for a stockbroker to get the experience I needed to stand out on my job application was a lot of work. How could I walk away now? I kept thinking maybe just doing what I was doing was not that bad. I wanted to stay in denial.

My perception at the time was that change would be more difficult. My expectations for change were not realistic. I felt like a victim, scared, and hopeless to create the change I needed to find a better work environment.

One day, my former husband said, "Let's go to a Tony Robbins firewalk conference." This was back in 1990. It was expensive, and I was reluctant. However, we both hated our jobs and felt stuck in the way we thought. My former husband had to also think about health insurance because of his type 1 diabetes.

For both of us, we felt the stress of showing up to a job we hated ultimately would impact our health. Stress can kill you. I knew it, but the denial was the easier way out.

If you are unfamiliar with Tony Robbins, he is a motivational speaker who teaches mind over matter, meaning your thoughts direct your actions. His approach was extremely novel at the time; all you had to do was walk over fire coals, and you would feel better. Yes, like the coals in your barbecue. It sounded ridiculous to me, but my former husband reminded me how much we both hated our jobs; that we had to keep moving forward until we found our way. He was right, and I knew it. I could pretend at work that everything was okay but not at home. There was a reason why many of my co-workers were having heart attacks. What I did not understand was why the people who had heart attacks came back to work so soon after a medical emergency, going against their healthcare providers' medical advice. I did not want that to be me.

A few days after the fire walk concept was introduced to me, I told my former husband I would go and participate in everything but the fire walk. But Tony must have been tuned into people like me who wanted to watch from the sidelines.

We got to the event. It was a three-day conference. Thousands of excited people showed up motivated about creating change in their lives. The fire walk was scheduled for the end of the evening of the first day. Tony explained that even if you did not want to walk over coals, you needed to stay in line, and when it was your turn, you could step out of line.

We left the conference hall late at night, winding our way outside onto a lawn with Tiki lights illuminating the road. Tony instructed us to chant, "Cool mas, cool mas." Imagine thousands of people in rows chanting "cool mas, cool mas" as they made their way down to the coals, excited about the experience.

My monkey brain became afraid that it is a cult event that I am getting sucked into at a vulnerable time in my life.

I broke my chant periodically as we headed to the hot coals, reminding my former husband that I had no intention of walking on them. He was supportive and told me all I had to do was walk over to the coals. Once it was my turn, I could step aside.

My turn came, and to my surprise, I decided to walk on the coals. As I walked, I remember thinking, "Oh my God! I cannot believe I am doing this!" But the minute I stopped my chant and had this one thought, I could feel a burn on my left foot near my arch. As an instinctive survival response, I started chanting "cool mas, cool mas" again, walking quickly over the coals to get to the other end.

Sugar Happy

After completing the fire walk, I felt exhilarated. Still doubting myself, I could not believe I had walked on hot coals. I went back to the coals, knelt down, and put my hand over them. They were hot.

I learned a lot that weekend about my limiting thoughts and what I can and cannot do. Most notably, we only create change in our lives for two reasons: to feel better or to stop feeling bad. Another important concept that I learned is, if you want to do something, like make a career change, don't reinvent the wheel. Study what successful people do and model it.

Creating change after a diabetes diagnosis requires a shift in the way you think. To illustrate this, I have two friends with husbands who were both diagnosed with type 2 diabetes and feared developing diabetes complications more than they feared lifestyle changes. After their diagnoses, they changed their lifestyles to avoid diabetes complications, knowing, in the long run, they would be happier.

My mother, brother, and aunt, all people who also had type 2 diabetes, felt more joy by being in denial about their diabetes until they started experiencing complications. My aunt passed away from a cardiovascular event. My mother was blind with cardiovascular disease and neuropathy. My brother, even after a cardiovascular event, could not wait to get out of the hospital to smoke a cigarette. A year after his hospital stay, he passed away.

There is no blame or shame here. It all boils down to feeling good or changing because you fear feeling bad later.

In my family's case, change felt like their happiness was being robbed. In the case of my friends' husbands, *not* changing felt like their happiness was going to be stolen. Same thought, both sides wanting to be happy with a different twist, two different outcomes - fatal or vital.

Working with Your Healthcare Professional Team

Over the years, I have had both good and bad experiences with healthcare professionals. No profession is immune to this. However, I want you to know that there are a lot of fantastic healthcare professionals who care about your diabetes success because they have seen the results of patients ignoring their diabetes. If you are working with someone you do not like and have the option of going to a different healthcare provider, don't doubt yourself. Diabetes success requires a team effort. Work with the people you want. It is of the utmost importance to see your healthcare professional team throughout the year to possibly impede or prevent complications that can be treated sooner than later. Your primary care physician will refer you to a specialist if necessary.

Let's *look* at who might be part of your diabetes healthcare team.

Primary Care Physician (PCP) — For some, this is the healthcare professional they will see for their regular checkups. The PCP may be your diabetes healthcare professional. Alternatively, the PCP may refer you to a specialist.

Sugar Happy

Endocrinologist — This is an endocrine system specialist who sees people with all kinds of endocrine disorders, including diabetes. Together you will set an A1c goal. Your A1c is the average blood sugar readings for the last three months. If your blood sugar is out of the prescribed range when checking with a glucose meter, you may want to reach out to your endocrinologist before your next scheduled visit. A quick phone consolation may help you sooner than later.

Nutritionist/Dietitian —This expert plays a vital role in helping you create a meal plan that will help you maintain a good blood glucose range. Your individualized meal plan can include suggestions for what to do when attending holiday, work, and family parties. It helps to have a strategy before you go to these events.

Eye Doctor— An optometrist can assess and diagnose diabetes-related eye problems, while an ophthalmologist is trained to diagnose and treat eye disease; treatment can include surgery.

Cardiologist —A heart surgeon and physician can ensure you do not have an artery obstruction, which is a possible complication of diabetes and high blood sugar levels.

Neurologist — It is important to regularly examine your nerves and nervous system to prevent or treat neuropathy, both central and peripheral neuropathy. Central neuropathy, like it sounds, is initiated in the central nervous system. There are many causes. Diabetes is just one possible cause.

Peripheral neuropathy affects the feelings in your hands and feet, diminishing your ability to feel or even to notice when you have hurt yourself. Peripheral neuropathy can happen when you have consistently high blood sugars due to diabetes, but just like central neuropathy, diabetes is only one of many possible causes.

Nephrologist — This kidney expert tests your kidney function to ensure the fluids that filter through the kidneys are normal.

Podiatrist — Regular examinations of your feet and ankles can ensure you do not have nerve damage, wounds, or infections. They can even make sure your toenails are cut properly and assist you in finding the best shoes to help prevent foot complications.

Diabetes Educator — One of my favorite healthcare professionals for people living with diabetes and one of your most essential resources. They can be doctors, pharmacists, nurses, or dietitians. A certified diabetes educator (CDE) is often your first stop when getting help to properly manage your diabetes.

In some states, nurse practitioners have the authority to diagnose diseases and prescribe medications for their patients. If you live in a state where your certified diabetes educator cannot diagnose or prescribe medications, they will work with your healthcare provider and pharmacist to ensure you have the proper medication you need to manage your diabetes. Some CDEs conduct diabetes support groups or will refer you to existing groups in your area.

Dentist — Diabetes has been shown to increase the risks of oral problems and diseases. A regular dental exam can even detect diabetes before you are diagnosed.

Sugar Happy

Make a Conscious Choice

Diabetes is called a silent killer. It is an invisible disease that can give you a false sense of comfort that everything is OK. Even if you take medications, if you don't change your diet or exercise, it may be only a matter of time before you start experiencing complications. It is like driving a stick shift car in first gear going 45 miles an hour. You can do it, but after a while, everything may start breaking down because you have overexerted the engine.

Consistently high blood sugars can cause changes in your organs. Being in denial after your diagnosis by not making any lifestyle changes, not testing your blood sugar, or taking medications without lowering your A1c to maintain a healthy range as defined by your healthcare professional, can cause diabetes complications. My mother once said to me, "If I knew it would be like this, I would have taken better care of myself." She was going blind and could no longer read. She had nerve damage. She was in constant pain. She suffered a heart attack. Clogged arteries and vascular surgery made her susceptible to blood clots. She went into a coma shortly after her vascular surgery and passed away at my home with the help of hospice.

This question is not meant to be judgmental in any way, but ask yourself, is this the quality of life you want for yourself?

What Does It Mean to Be in Denial?

Some people think taking their medication is all they have to do in managing their diabetes. It is much more complicated than that.

Testing your blood sugar is imperative, regardless of if you take medication or not. Knowing where your blood sugar level lies helps you make better decisions with your diet and exercise. A close friend of mine was recently diagnosed with type 2 diabetes. They visited me one day for lunch. Before eating, they tested their blood sugar. It was high. They decided to delay eating and opted to go for a walk to bring down their blood sugar.

Years ago, in one of my children's classes, I met a father who had had type 1 diabetes. To my surprise, he did not have a blood glucose meter despite having had type 1 for over 10 years. I asked him, "How do you know how much insulin to take after eating if you do not check your blood sugar?"

"I guess," he said.

Later, I found out from other parents who knew him better than I did, that guessing his blood sugar kept him on a chronically hypoglycemic (low blood sugar) roller coaster ride. As we got to know each other better, he eventually got a blood glucose meter and started testing. As a result, he did not have as many low blood sugar episodes that he had to treat from his "guessing" game.

Lifestyle Changes You Need to Make

Quit smoking. Statistically, if you have diabetes and smoke, you have a higher percentage of having a kidney, heart, and blood vessel disease. Unfortunately, my brother who passed away at the age of 53, illustrates this point.

Sugar Happy

If you have diabetes and take insulin, smoking also affects your insulin dosing, making it challenging to maintain healthy blood sugar levels.

Lose excess weight and exercise. Some people may be able to decrease the medications they are taking or even stop taking them altogether once they lose excess weight and start exercising. Then, there is the added benefit of how well they feel and the applause they get from family and friends. If you have lost weight, your medications may need to be adjusted, but do not do this on your own. Work with your healthcare provider.

Lower your high blood pressure. It puts pressure on your body's organs and can lead to blood vessel damage, kidney disease, stroke, even heart attacks, among other conditions.

Prevent high blood sugars. Hyperglycemia may affect your ability to see, causing you to lose feeling in your feet, affect your kidneys, and even cause the ultimate complication of losing your life.

The Impact of Lifestyle Changes

Once you look at your habits, you will be surprised at how the small tweaks you make in your diet and exercise can make a big difference. Today, we have so many food choices to replace our favorite comfort foods. We know a lot more about nutrition and what drives us to eat. So, take a stance. Are you eating to live or living to eat?

Living to eat means you love indulging in food. It is always on your mind; you cannot wait to eat something because it is going to make you happy. The Mayo Clinic describes emotional eating as events in our lives that trigger eating foods when we feel stressed. It is a coping mechanism that sabotages weight loss and can contribute to excess weight.

Eating to live is when you are aware of your nutritional needs and what is best for your body to manage or avoid disease.

Chances are, a genetic predisposition, such as having a family history of type 2 diabetes, smoking, excess weight, or some other undetermined variable led to your diabetes diagnosis. In some cases, certain medications can contribute to excess weight or maybe diabetes is even listed as a possible side effect of a medication you are taking to treat a different medical issue. Whatever the cause, you can learn more about how to control the things you can and use lifestyle changes to bring about a better outcome for your diabetes management and your health overall.

Your Personal Take Away Notes To Remember

CHAPTER 3

UNDERSTANDING HOW MEDICATIONS WORK

Drug therapy is available for both type 1 and type 2 diabetes. If you have type 1, insulin is a requirement. There are a variety of insulins on the market. If you have type 2 diabetes and cannot successfully manage it with diet and exercise alone, medication therapy would most likely start with metformin. Insulin therapy is just as much an option for people with type 2 as it is for people with type 1. Despite the misconception, needing insulin is not a sign of failure or an indication that your type 2 diabetes is getting worse. No two people with diabetes are the same, so what works for each person won't necessarily be the same either. The medications you use will depend on your specific treatment plan and blood glucose target that you set up as a goal with your healthcare team.

Type 2 Oral Medications

There are many type 2 medications on the market, both oral and injectable. These medications are broken down by classification and how they function internally. For example, some type 2 medications will stimulate the pancreas to make insulin while others will prevent starches from turning into sugar to prevent high blood sugar. Below, these medications are broken down by class, including the **Brand name** (generic) for each medication. This list is by no means exhaustive as some classes also include combination medications.

Medications are being added and subtracted all the time as studies and trials continue to prove or disprove their effectiveness. Always talk with your prescribing healthcare professional about the benefits and side effects of any medications that are included in your treatment plan. For added measure, double-check with your pharmacist as well, to ensure that the different active prescriptions do not have a negative impact, making the therapy inadvisable.

Alpha-glucosidase Inhibitors

These starch blockers work in the intestines to slow down the digestion of some carbohydrates so that after-meal blood glucose peaks are not so high.

Medications currently include:

- **Glyset** (miglitol)
- **Precose** (acarbose)

Possible side effects include abdominal pain, gas, and diarrhea.

Sugar Happy

Biguanides

Better known as metformin, these commonly used type 2 medications work by reducing the liver's glucose production.

Medications currently include:

- **Fortamet** (metformin extended-release)
- **Glucophage** (metformin)
- **Glucophage XR** (metformin extended-release)
- **Glumetza** (metformin extended-release)

Possible side effects include bloating, diarrhea, gas, heartburn, lower back or side pain, and upset stomach; but the most common (and commonly desired) side effect is decreased appetite.

Dopamine D_2 Receptor Agonist

In people with type 2 diabetes, dopamine activity in the brain is believed to be too low in the morning about waking time. Morning Cycloset increases dopamine activity in the brain at this time. More normal dopamine activity in the brain at this time of day may help one's body more effectively use insulin to move glucose from the blood into tissues to be used immediately as energy or stored for later use. Taken daily in the morning was shown to lower blood sugar levels after each meal of the day without raising plasma insulin levels. Over time, this may help one reach their A1c goal.

Possible side effects include gastrointestinal distress, hypertension, dizziness when rising from a sitting position, and may exacerbate existing psychotic disorders.

Bile acid sequestrants (BAS)

These medications were initially and successfully used to lower cholesterol, but then studies began to show that they also improved glycemic control in people with type 2 diabetes when used in conjunction with metformin, sulfonylureas, or insulin. There is currently only one FDA- approved BAS:

- **Welchol** (colesevelam)

Possible side effects include raised triglyceride (blood fat) levels and may cause constipation, stomach upset, low blood sugar, and high blood pressure.

Dipeptidyl peptidase-4 inhibitors (DPP-4)

Also called "gliptins," DPP-4 medications prevent the breakdown of GLP-1 (See Injectable (Non-Insulin) Medications below) thus increasing your insulin level and lowering blood sugar.

Medications currently include:

- **Januvia** (sitagliptin)
- **Nesina** (alogliptin)
- **Onglyza** (saxagliptin)
- **Tradjenta** (linagliptin)

Sugar Happy

Possible side effects include upper respiratory tract infections, headaches, skin rash, facial swelling, and urinary tract infections (mostly linked to taking saxagliptin).

Gastrointestinal symptoms, such as diarrhea and nausea, may occur, too.

These medicines have been linked with an increased risk for pancreatitis

Meglitinides

Meglitinides stimulate the pancreas to produce more insulin quickly and must be timed with meals to avoid low blood sugar. They work the same as sulfonylureas (see below) but have a shorter duration of effectiveness.

Medications currently include:

- **Prandin** (repaglinide)
- **Starlix** (nateglinide)

Possible side effects include hypoglycemia, headache, nasal congestion, weight gain, and less commonly, constipation, diarrhea, upper respiratory infection, and back pain.

Sodium Glucose Transporter 2 (SGLT2)

SGLT2 work by removing the sugar through urine and preventing the kidney from absorbing sugar.

Medications currently include:

- **Farxiga** (dapagliflozin)
- **Invokana** (canagliflozin)
- **Jardiance** (empagliflozin)
- **Steglatro** (ertugliflozin)
- **Synjardy** (empagliozin and metformin hydrochloride)

Possible side effects include urinary tract and genital infections, dehydration (due to increased urination)

Sulfonylureas

As with the meglitinides class above, sulfonylureas work by stimulating the pancreas to make more insulin. (Interesting side note: This is the oldest of all the classes of diabetes medications, having first been developed in the 1940s.)

Medications currently include:

- **Amaryl** (glimepiride)
- **DiaBeta** (glyburide)
- **Diabinese** (chlorpropamide)
- **GlipZIDE XL** (glipizide)
- **Glucotrol** (glipizide)
- **Glucotrol XL** (glipizide extended-release)
- **Glycron** (glyburide)
- **Glynase** (glyburide)

- **Micronase** (glyburide)
- **Tol-Tab** (tolbutamide)
- **Tolinase** (Pro)

Possible side effects include hypoglycemia and weight gain. Less common side effects are skin rash and upset stomach.

Thiazolidinediones (TZDs)

TZDs work by increasing insulin sensitivity in the muscles and fat cells.

They also lower glucose production. Medications currently include:

- **Actos** (pioglitazone)
- **Avandia** (rosiglitazone)

Possible side effects include hypoglycemia, edema, fluid retention (which increases the risk for or may worsen heart failure), weight gain.

Injectable (Non-Insulin) Medications

Amylin Mimetic

This injectable medication slows food movement through the stomach. Blood sugar is then prevented from rising too high following a meal, which may make you feel fuller and maybe even cause weight loss. It works with insulin to lower blood sugars.

- **Symlin** (pramlintide)

Possible side effects include an increased risk of hypoglycemia due to the timing of premeal insulin in conjunction with delayed food absorption. Also, stomach pain, fatigue, dizziness, cough, sore throat, and joint pain.

Glucagon-like peptide-1 receptor agonist (GLP-1)

GLP-1 causes the pancreas to make insulin when blood sugar levels are too high. It also slows down digestion, causing a decrease in appetite. Also known as incretin mimetics, these drugs work best with diet and exercise.

- **Adlyxin** (lixisenatide)
- **Bydureon/Bydurean BCise** (exenatide extended-release)
- **Byetta** (exenatide)
- **Eperzan** (albiglutide)
- **Ozempic** (semaglutide)
- **Soliqua** (lixisenatide)
- **Tanzeum** (albiglutide)
- **Trulicty** (dulaglutide)
- **Victoza** (liraglutide)

Possible side effects include changes in blood sugar, nausea, and occasionally, vomiting, followed by diarrhea/constipation.

Insulin Types and How Long They Take to Work

Like oral medications, the effectiveness of insulin therapy varies. But before explaining the specific types of insulin, it is crucial to

47

understand that they all fall into one of two categories – basal or bolus.

Known as background insulin, basal insulin covers the long-acting and intermediate categories. This insulin keeps the blood glucose consistent during periods of fasting.

Bolus insulin is primarily taken at mealtimes, thus covering the rapid- acting and short-acting categories. It can also be used to correct highs in blood sugar levels.

The most common side effect of any insulin therapy is a low blood glucose (hypoglycemia), so be sure to keep a check on your numbers.

Rapid-Acting Insulin

This insulin is usually taken pre-meal and used with long-acting insulin. It is also used to correct blood sugar highs. While most of these insulins start working 10–20 minutes after you inject, a couple of them begin sooner after injecting. They stay in the system 1.5–5 hours, depending on the insulin.

- **Admelog** (insulin lispro)
- **Afrezza** (inhalation powder)
- **Apidra** (insulin glulisine U-100)
- **Fiasp** (insulin aspart U-100)
- **Humalog** (insulin lispro U-100/U-200)
- **NovoLog** (insulin aspart U-100)

Short-Acting Insulin

Usually taken about 30 minutes before eating, this insulin is typically used with long-acting insulin. It starts working 30–60 minutes after injection and stays in the system for 5–8 hours.

- **Humulin R** (regular U 100/U-500)
- **Novolin R** (regular U-100/U500)
- **ReliOn Novolin R** (regular U-100)

Intermediate-Acting Insulin

When rapid-acting insulin ceases to work, intermediate-acting can step in. It is usually used with rapid-acting or short-acting and taken twice a day. It starts working 1–3 hours after you inject and stay in your system 12–24 hours.

- **Humulin N** (NPH U-100)
- **Novolin N** (NPH U-100)
- **ReliOn Novolin R** (NPH U-100)

Long-Acting Insulin

Taken once or twice a day, long-acting kicks in when rapid-acting insulin stops working. It can also be used with short-acting insulin.

This insulin starts working in the system 1–1.6 hours after injection and stays in the system up to 24 hours.

- **Basaglar** (insulin glargine U-100)
- **Lantus** (insulin glargine U-100)

Sugar Happy

- **Levemir** (insulin detemir U-100)
- **Soliqua** (insulin glargine 100/33 U100)
- **Tresbia** (insulin degludec U100/U200)
- **Toujeo** (insulin glargine U300)
- **Xultophy** (insulin degludec 100/3.6 U100)

Ultra-Long-Acting Insulin

This insulin starts working in the system after 1–16 hours and stays in the system for up to 36–42 hours.

- **Toujeo** (insulin glargine U-300)
- **Tresiba** (insulin degludec U-100/U-200)

Intermediate Rapid-Acting Insulin

This category of insulin consists of insulin mixtures that start working 10–20 minutes after injection and stay in the system for 16–24 hours.

- **Humalog Mix 50/50** (50% lispro protamine (NPL)/50% insulin lispro U-100)
- **Humalog Mix 75/25** (75% lispro protamine (NPL)/25% insulin lispro U-100)
- **Novolog Mix 70/30** (70% aspart protamine/30% insulin aspart U- 100)

Intermediate Short-Acting Insulin

These are also insulin mixtures. They start working 30–60 minutes after injection and stay in the system from 12–24 hours.

- **Humulin 70/30** (70% NPH/30% Regular U-100)
- **Novolin 70/30** (70% NPH/30% Regular U-100)

Don't Fear Insulin

People with type 2 diabetes fear using syringes, thus, delaying insulin, and GLP- 1 medication that may offer superior glycemic control when other drugs fail them. The thought of injecting may make your heart race, cause dizziness, or get you sweaty. We call this needle phobia. The image of turning away from a large hospital syringe and bracing yourself for the pain can also contribute to your phobia.

For type 1, you do not have the option of delaying injections; insulin is crucial to living. Going on an insulin pump, inserting a canula (soft needle connected to an infusion set) once every three days can be more attractive than daily multiple injections. Talk with her healthcare provider about which treatment is most suitable for your lifestyle.

Overcoming the Injecting Barrier

When I had my diabetes supply store and spoke to insulin-dependent type 1s and type 2s who had overcome their needle phobia, they shared how surprised they were by how much more painful it was to lance their finger for a blood glucose check than it was for them to take an insulin injection. The reason being syringes have come a long way. The size of the needle is much smaller now, giving people many options depending on their personal needs. Lancets have also evolved to be less painful than 30 years ago.

I wanted to walk a mile in a pump wearer's shoes. I decided to put myself on an insulin pump with saline and a bent needle for a week to get a first-hand experience of what it was like to wear a pump daily. Inserting the needle was the biggest hurdle for me, but once I did it successfully, my confidence skyrocketed. Wearing an insulin pump helped me understand issues like my tubing getting caught on a door handle, putting the pump underneath the pillow when sleeping, wearing clothes to accommodate my pump. The simple act of getting dressed was much more complicated than I realized. Every day, I had to decide where to put my insulin pump as I was getting dressed. The tubing needed to be long enough to put the insulin pump on my chest of drawers or the bed as I put on my pants.

Other methods for insulin injection, such as using a device that injects the insulin, masking the injection process, so you don't see or feel the needle is helpful for some.

There are creams on the market that numb the area before you inject, requiring planning as you wait for the cream to take effect. The old school way is to put ice on an area before injecting. Some people say this helps with minimizing the pain.

Another barrier to taking injections is the fear of taking insulin, worrying that you cannot handle giving yourself an injection or that you might get a low blood sugar. Unfortunately, this also reduces one's adherence, meaning taking injections less frequently than you are supposed to, preventing you from achieving optimal blood sugar levels.

My mother went on insulin. She did overcome her needle phobia. But she was scared to correct her high blood sugar reading, especially if her blood glucose test showed a reading of 180 mg/dL. In most cases, her blood sugar test results were between 240mg/dL to 350 mg/dL. Had she worked more closely with her healthcare professional, she could have learned how many units of insulin to take, to attain her ideal glucose threshold. Learn how many units you need to bring down a high blood sugar, it is all a learning process.

My brother checked his blood sugar infrequently when he lived in Australia. Once he came to visit me, he went on insulin and started checking his blood sugar more frequently. His success came from being diabetes literate. He learned the importance of diet, medication, and checking his blood sugar.

If you find injecting insulin or a type 2 medication scary, there are many ways to overcome your insulin injection fears. Work with your healthcare team. They are skilled in helping you overcome your needle phobia by being on the lookout for devices and methods to assist you in making your therapy easier.

Sugar Happy

How to Manage Your Blood Sugar

The purpose of managing your blood sugar is to maintain a consistent target blood glucose target range and to delay or prevent diabetes complications. It is of the utmost importance to work with your healthcare professional team to learn which diet plan is best for you, which exercise program is more suitable for you, the best routine for daily blood glucose checks, and how to take your medications regularly.

Learning how to bring down a high blood sugar or bring up a low blood sugar will give you confidence in managing your diabetes. Like anything new, it may seem overwhelming at first, but the daily practice of diabetes self- management will provide you with a better outcome than ignoring your diabetes. Denial predictably will lower the quality of your life and deprive loved ones of having you there during their milestones in life.

My mother, for example, classified her diabetes as having a good day or bad day, meaning she watched her diet, exercised, and took her medication (a good day), or she ate what she wanted regardless of her diabetes (a bad day). She would say things like "I was a good girl" or "I was a bad girl." She vacillated between taking care of her diabetes and being in denial.

I had many conversations with her, explaining that blood glucose management requires the integration of being diabetes literate and taking her medication as prescribed. I demonstrated how to use her medical devices so they could tell her what she needed to know. We discussed diet, exercise, and staying hydrated to delay or prevent diabetes complications. She was not motivated to understand her diabetes until she started experiencing complications from high blood sugar. She passed away at 65, which was a significant loss to my family.

Diabetes is called a silent killer because you think you are fine, but internally, the damage is occurring when you have high blood sugar. Just because you cannot see it, does not mean your internal organs are functioning optimally.

I still miss my mother and brother. What is the one thing they both taught me?

Ignoring your health has irreversible consequences.

In the end, the loss of a loved one is more painful than you realize for the people you leave behind.

Know Your A1c

The A1c—sometimes referred to as the Hemoglobin A1c, glycosylated hemoglobin, glycated Hemoglobin, and HbA1c—measures your average glucose from 60 to 90 days. When you check your blood sugar with a blood glucose meter, it only tells you what your glucose level is at that moment in time. It does not accurately reflect all the highs and lows you experience, nor does it indicate the direction your blood glucose could be trending.

Sugar Happy

Blood cells form and die within 90 days. The A1c test records the memory in the blood, giving us an average reading that correlates with the percentage.

Sometimes you can get a false A1c level if you have anemia, an iron deficiency, a blood transfusion, or a plethora of other reasons.

The percentage can also vary depending on where you get your A1C checked. So, it is best to use the same lab if possible.

A1c Target Goals

The American Diabetes Association (ADA) recommends checking your A1c at least twice a year. Their recommended target A1C varies. For most adults who are not pregnant, the recommended target is <7% (53 mmol/mol).

A tighter goal of <6.5% (48 mmol/mol) is recommended for select patients, including:

- people who are newly diagnosed
- people with type 2 that is treated with lifestyle changes or metformin only
- people with a long-life expectancy
- people with no significant cardiovascular disease.

Conversely, the ADA recommends a looser A1c target of <8% (64 mmol/mol) for select people:

- People with a history of severe hypoglycemia
- people with a limited life expectancy

- people with advanced microvascular or macrovascular complications
- People diagnosed with an extensive amount of other conditions
- People who have had diabetes for a long time and who have difficulty achieving their target despite ongoing efforts

The American Association of Clinical Endocrinologists (AACE) recommends setting a target based on the person's age, other diseases they may be living with, and how long they have had diabetes.

For most people, they recommend an A1c target of ≤6.5, but for healthier people, a tighter goal closer to normal (below 5.7%) is suggested. For people who are not as healthy, a looser A1c target is recommended.

The United Kingdom Prospective Diabetes Study (UKPDS) researched newly diagnosed patients with type 2 diabetes over a 10-year period, exploring tight glucose management through diet, type 2 medications and insulin.

The patient with tight control who was under intensive management with an A1c of 7 experienced a 25% reduction in possible damage to the eye, kidney, and nerve. Additionally, for every 1% reduction in the patient's A1c, there was a 21% decrease in diabetes complications.

In the United States, a landmark Diabetes Control and Complications Study for people with type 1 diabetes also demonstrated that tight glucose control reduced diabetes complications.

The Science Behind the A1c

Hemoglobin is a protein located inside the red blood cells. Oxygen molecules bind to the hemoglobin molecules, allowing oxygen to be delivered to the cells of the body.

The sugar in your body binds or glycates to the hemoglobin. The higher the amount of sugar, the more hemoglobin gets glycated. The A1c measures this glycated hemoglobin and gives you an average over the past 2 to 3 months. If the glycated hemoglobin is high, it limits the oxygen delivery, which is when vascular complications can occur.

Work with your healthcare team to set a target A1c. Understanding the importance of your A1c, taking your medication, watching your diet, exercising, checking your blood sugar, staying hydrated, and continuously working to lower your A1c can all work together to prevent diabetes complications.

Time and Range Versus A1C

Your healthcare professional might start using the term "time and range" instead of A1c. The significance is that this new measurement looks at how long your blood sugar stays within a certain range while the A1c provides you with the average blood sugar for 90 days. Knowing how long your blood sugar stays at a certain range can help your healthcare professional fine-tune your therapy and or medication, possibly allowing you to experience fewer highs and lows in your routine care.

Your Personal Take Away Notes To Remember

CHAPTER 4

WHY MAINTAINING NORMAL BLOOD SUGARS IS IMPORTANT TO AVOIDING COMPLICATIONS

Diabetes is when your body is unable to balance the sugar level in your bloodstream. High blood sugar affects every part of your body because the sugar is converted into energy, driving the functions of your organs. The manufactured glucose carries the energy through the bloodstream. It either helps you function correctly by maintaining the biochemical balance your body needs, or it hurts normal function, creating health issues that show up as diabetes complications.

Prolonged high blood sugar imbalance hurts the natural function of your organs. It can affect the eyes, kidney, heart, nerves, skin, feet, and can even lead to periodontal disease.

Sugar Happy

When you eat starch or sugar, the food in your stomach breaks down into glucose, which is released into your bloodstream. Your pancreas then releases insulin to convert the sugar into energy in your cells. Insulin is the key needed to open the blood cells so they can either use the sugar as energy or store it. If your pancreas does not release enough insulin to transport the sugar into your blood cells, the excess sugar stays in your bloodstream, giving you a high blood sugar reading. This makes your organs work harder to expel the extra sugar. If it remains in your bloodstream for long periods, it can start affecting your nerves and organs.

Keeping your blood sugar levels in a healthy range is important to preventing diabetes complications.

Common Diabetes Complications Retinopathy

The retina is the back part of the eye that translates images through impulses to the brain, signaling us to do something or stop what we are doing. For example, if you are driving a car and see an accident ahead, your brain will alert your muscles to slow down by placing your foot on the brake and pressing down to slow or stop the car.

According to the National Eye Institute, diabetic eye disease increased in prevalence by 89 percent between 2000 and 2010 and is a leading cause of blindness among American adults. Despite this, people with diabetes often overlook vision care as they work to manage the many other health problems the disease can cause.

Why Maintaining Normal Blood Sugars Is Important

My mother went blind from her chronic high blood sugar, making her homecare more complicated. I managed her daily thyroid, blood pressure, cholesterol, depression and insulin injections while raising a 3 - and 5-year-old and running my business. I did this willingly and with love. My mother brought me into this world, the natural cycle for me was to be there for her when she was ready to leave this world.

Her vision checkups were irregular. Like most people, she assumed some of her vision fluctuations were a result of her aging. She never connected diabetes and retinopathy.

A survey conducted by the American Optometric Association demonstrates eye disease may not have symptoms for people living with diabetes, possibly causing it to go undiagnosed. Additionally, many Americans do not know that a person with diabetes should have a comprehensive eye exam once a year, including a retina (dilated) eye exam.

These exams are the only way to diagnose serious eye diseases in their early stages that are associated with diabetes. Progressive eye diseases often begin without warning.

The longer a person has diabetes, the higher the chances of an eye disease. Over time, diabetes may cause damage to the blood vessels in the back of the eye, a condition known as diabetic retinopathy, which can lead to diabetic macular edema (DME). DME occurs when the damaged blood vessels leak fluid and cause swelling. Although symptoms are not always present, this swelling can cause blurred vision, double vision, floaters, or black or white space.

Getting regular checkups to catch potential complications before they worsen is why you should never skip your eye appointment.

What is more important than keeping your sight? Nothing!

Treatment for Retinopathy

If you have mild or moderate retinopathy, immediate treatment may not be required. Working with your healthcare provider to maintain a good blood sugar range may slow down the progression.

Proliferative retinopathy requires laser surgery to cauterize (burn) leaking blood vessels and reduce the swelling in the eye.

Corticosteroids are another therapy using implants or injections in the eye, possibly in conjunction with other medications and laser surgery, to treat the disease.

Nephrology

The purpose of the kidneys is to first filter out compounds from our body that it does not need, releasing them through urination. It then reabsorbs compounds we do need through further filtration of the blood before the rest goes back into our bloodstream.

Kahn Academy explains that our two kidneys retain 22% of our body's blood supply and can filter all our blood in five minutes. The two million filters known as nephrons do these 400 times a day.

Why Maintaining Normal Blood Sugars Is Important

Kidney damage occurs when high blood sugar affects the filtration of the kidneys by stretching the small blood cells known as capillaries. The constant ongoing stress to the kidney capillaries eventually causes the kidneys to fail.

The National Kidney Foundation reports that people with diabetes have a 1.3 % chance of experiencing kidney disease, identifying it as the #1 cause of kidney failure.

Eating a diet high in salt will affect the kidneys' filtration by disturbing the natural balance, creating high blood pressure. Drinking the suggested 64 ounces of water daily helps with the metabolic filtration process.

Alcohol obstructs the tubular filtration, putting you at risk for kidney disease.

Caffeine and chocolate can raise your blood pressure, which also stresses the kidney filtration system.

Smoking cigarettes narrow the blood vessels, reducing the blood flow.

Kidney care starts with watching your blood sugars and watching your diet. Eliminate foods and drinks that restrict the filtration so that your body's balance is not disrupted, decreasing your chance of being diagnosed with kidney disease.

Treatment for Nephrology

You may be asked to watch your diet, lose weight if need be, cut out tobacco and alcohol. There is a school of thought that a

---

lower protein diet is preferred but speak to your healthcare provider first.

A small rise in blood pressure can stress your kidney function, so controlling your blood pressure may be recommended.

If you do reach the end stage of kidney disease, dialysis, and kidney transplantation are the common treatment options.

Neuropathy

Neuropathy is a loss nerve function. High blood sugars can affect the nervous system, impacting the ability to feel and respond accordingly. The result is nerve damage. High blood sugars bind to the protein in the arteries, obstructing the blood flow and damaging the nerves. Think of the texture of turkey jerky; this is what happens when your arteries have high blood sugars flowing through them.

Let's say you are reaching over a stovetop, and a burner is on, but you did not see it. The healthy nerves in your hand that come close to the heat will send a nerve impulse to your brain at what seems like the speed of light, and your brain will send an impulse down your spinal cord to the nerves in your hand, alerting you to the danger. The physical response will be to pull away from the burner or to be aware of the potential threat of getting hurt.

If you have sensory neuropathy, the nerves in your hand may not be able to feel the heat or send the signal to your brain and back again, causing you to burn yourself.

People with diabetes more commonly have polyneuropathy, which is a general degeneration of the nerves. There can be loss of sensation in their hands and feet, inability to detect pain, failure to detect temperature, twitching, muscle weakness, pain, intolerance to heat, lack of bladder control, constipation, diarrhea, impaired breathing, and reduced heart rate.

The Mayo Clinic estimates that at least 50% of people with diabetes experience some type of neuropathy.

Treatment for Neuropathy

Medication for neuropathy includes anti-inflammatory drugs, painkillers, anti-seizure drugs, antidepressants, and topical creams.

Physical therapy may also help increase your muscle movement.

Foot Care

It is of the utmost importance to pay attention to your feet, especially if you have neuropathy. Little things like calluses and corns should be removed by a healthcare professional to avoid potential infection. Don't use any sharp foot care products to take care of these minor foot irritations at home.

The Centers for Disease Control and Prevention reports that foot ulcerations can become a gateway to infections, giving people with neuropathy a higher probability of getting a foot ulcer. Preventive care goes a long way.

Sugar Happy

Here are some ways you can take care of your feet.

- Don't walk barefoot, not even in your own home. You may step on something and not notice or feel it until it turns into an infection. For people with diabetes, the healing process can be slower. At its worst, an infection can turn into an amputation. With a visit to a healthcare professional, a small foot injury can be taken care of and healed.

- Before putting shoes on, check for objects like pebbles or hard spots that might create skin irritation while you are walking. Always wear socks, preferably without seams, for better blood flow.

- File your nails if you can. Use a hand mirror to help you see better, but if you notice any discoloration on your nails or a fungus or you are unable to trim your nails safely, make an appointment with your podiatrist.

- When bathing, check the temperature before you get in. It should be 90-95°F. Some healthcare professionals recommend using your elbow to gauge the heat of the water. If the water is too hot, it can damage your skin. If you soak your feet too long, it will dry your skin, potentially leading to wounds.

- Always pat your feet after they are washed and make sure the in-between areas of your toes are dry. Put cream on the top and bottom of your feet but not in between your toes. You want to avoid moisture in between the toes.

It is recommended to get a foot checkup annually. But people with diabetes and neuropathy should go every three months. It is better to catch an infection or lesion earlier because more treatment options will be available.

Treatment for Ulcers

A foot ulcer is an open sore or wound. If you develop an ulcer, there are several treatment options available, including but not limited to the following:

- Debridement of the wound, which is the removal of debris from the wound and the cutting away of unhealthy tissue. Assuming the foot has good tissue remaining for healthy blood circulation, debridement should stimulate the area to promote healing once again.

- Surgery or a procedure that diverts blood from the ulcer. This more advanced treatment may be necessary if the ulcer does not respond to initial treatment measures.

- Devices such as a removable cast to protect the tissue cell and limbs with a rocking design to prevent you from putting weight on the ulcer. This is called off-loading. A half shoe is the second choice for people who do not like the rocking device in the cast.

Skin Care

People with diabetes are more susceptible to bacterial and fungal infections than people without diabetes. Poor circulation and nerve damage narrow the blood vessels near the skin, possibly clogging it, preventing wounds from healing because of the lack of blood flow.

Dry skin associated with high blood sugars can increase vulnerability to bacterial infections. So, check your skin regularly for anything abnormal. Look for changes, such as an outbreak of spots, small red spots or otherwise; skin discoloration, red-brown or yellow skin tags, a thickness of the skin, foot ulcers, rashes, and blisters.

Treatment for Skin Care Issues

Preventive care is always the first recommendation.

- Use antibacterial soap when bathing to prevent an infection.
- Use skin cream daily. Buy a rich cream for those extra dry spots. Remember not to use cream between your toes, as avoiding moisture there prevents bacterial infection.

Dental Care

Bad breath and dry mouth can be related to diabetes. Sometimes new medications can give people bad breath. There are over 500 drugs and steroids that treat high blood pressure, cardiovascular heart disease, mental health, and allergies. Any number of these can yield foul mouth odor. Whether you have type 1 or type 2 diabetes, experiencing persistent bad breath and dry mouth can be a warning that is not to be ignored. High blood sugar does play a role in the process.

Why Maintaining Normal Blood Sugars Is Important

Halitosis

Commonly referred to as bad breath, halitosis can be a result of high blood sugar. This occurs when bacteria mix with the plaque on your teeth. When you eat a meal, particles of the food usually stay in your mouth. Bacteria feed on the sugar from the food particles in your mouth and releases a bad smell.

High blood sugar is a breeding ground for bacteria and causes bad breath. There are over 700 bacteria strains in our mouths. While most are good, others can be harmful and contribute to gum disease.

If the bacteria and plaque go unattended, you will be at risk for periodontal gum disease. Of all the people diagnosed with diabetes, 22% have gum disease.

Xerostomia

Saliva helps with the digestion process by allowing us to taste and digest food. Saliva also neutralizes the acid from food particles and prevents infections. The absence of saliva keeps your teeth and gums dry, allowing bacteria to flourish in developing cavities. This dry mouth condition is known as xerostomia, which can cause bad breath. Bleeding gums from dry mouth puts you at risk for gingivitis, the first stage of gum disease.

Alcohol-based mouthwashes are not recommended for people with dry mouth. But if you have diabetes and do not have dry mouth, then using a mouthwash with alcohol is shown to be the preferred treatment for oral health.

Sugar Happy

Treatment for Dental Issues

Oral health plays a significant role in preventing gum disease. Simple routines such as eating less sugar or starchy foods that turn to sugar, brushing and flossing your teeth after meals, using mouthwash to kill bacteria, and regular dental checkups will keep your teeth intact, treat bad breath and dry mouth, and contribute to a beautiful smile.

Don't miss your dental checkups. They can help save your gums and teeth.

Heart Care

Diabetes increases your chance of having heart disease, making you more susceptible to hypertension and elevated cholesterol. Maintaining blood sugars in the normal range can lower your risk of strokes and heart attacks.

If you have cardiovascular disease in your family, smoke cigarettes, have high blood pressure, elevated cholesterol, or have obesity, you are at a higher risk for cardiovascular disease.

My mother had cardiovascular disease, high blood pressure, and high cholesterol. She did not like the side effects of her blood pressure medication and took matters into her own hands — she stopped taking her drugs. To my dismay, she did not check in with her healthcare provider to explore her options. Shortly after her new, self-prescribed therapy, she had her first stroke.

Why Maintaining Normal Blood Sugars Is Important

Types of Cardiovascular Disease

Because of the high rate of high cholesterol and high blood pressure among people with diabetes, the risk of developing heart disease is significantly increased. It is the number one complication diagnosed among people with diabetes. According to the American Heart Association, adults with diabetes are two to four times more likely to die from heart disease than adults without diabetes. At least 68 percent of people who are age 65 or older and who have diabetes will die from some form of heart disease.

But it's not as simple as having a "heart problem." Like many things, heart diseases vary. Some of the most common heart diseases include:

- Coronary heart disease, which is when plaque (fat, cholesterol, calcium, and other substances found in the blood) builds up in your arteries, narrowing the blood flow. Arteries are the blood vessels carrying oxygen and nutrients, pushing substances up and down the body. At its worst, when the blood flow is clogged, a person will experience a heart attack.

- Congestive heart failure is when your heart has a difficult time pumping oxygen and blood in and out. Over time, coronary artery disease (a disease of the arteries) and even ongoing high blood pressure can leave your heart in a weakened state, which can lead to congestive heart failure.

- Peripheral artery disease is when there is a plaque buildup in the arteries, which narrows the blood flow from your arms and legs.
- Carotid artery disease is when there is a plaque in the arteries that supply blood to the brain.

Eating a healthy diet, lowering your blood pressure, decreasing your cholesterol, quitting smoking, and exercising are great preventive measures to reduce your risk for cardiovascular disease.

Treatment for Heart Care

A heart disease diagnosis is not necessarily a worst-case scenario. There are still treatment options available depending on the disease.

Surgeries

- Angioplasty is a procedure used to restore arterial blood flow. A small tube with a balloon at its end is temporarily inserted through your groin to get to the clogged area in your heart. Dye that is visible through X-ray is used to see the blockage. The balloon is then expanded inside the narrow arteries. If needed, a wire mesh called a stent is left in place to keep the treated area unobstructed.
- Cardioversion is a procedure used for irregular heartbeats, using electrical currents to reset the heart rhythm.
- Enhanced external counterpulsation (EECP) is a treatment that increases blood flow from the lower extremities through

a pressurized cuff, causing blood to travel from the limbs to the areas of the heart that need it.

- Heart bypass surgery is a procedure that graphs healthy arteries to a blocked artery in the heart.
- A heart transplant is when a diseased heart is replaced with a healthy donor heart, and the major blood vessels from the weak heart are attached to the new donor heart.
- A pacemaker and implantable cardioverter-defibrillator are devices used to regulate the heartbeat of people who suffer from arrhythmia, which is an irregular heartbeat.
- Valve disease treatment is when one or more of your four heart valves does not function properly. There are two therapies, a mechanical valve or a tissue valve aids in restoring natural blood flow to the four heart chambers.
- A left ventricular assist device is used when a heart cannot pump blood adequately. Usually used at the end stage of heart disease and while waiting for a transplant, it aids in pumping the blood in and out of your heart.

Medications

- Ace Inhibitors allow the blood vessels to enlarge and reduces blood pressure.
- Angiotensin II receptor blockers dilate the blood vessels, reducing blood pressure.
- Antiarrhythmics block the irregular heartbeat.

- Antiplatelets prevent blood clots.
- Aspirin is also an anti-clotting medication that is used to prevent strokes, a blood clot that travels to the brain.
- Beta-blockers block adrenaline to slow down the heart.
- Calcium channel blockers reduce the heartbeat and dilate the blood vessels.
- Clot buster drugs are used to prevent strokes by preventing the blood from clotting and traveling to the brain.
- Digoxin slows down the rate of the heartbeat.
- Diuretics stimulate the kidney to release salt and water through urine.
- Nitrates increase blood pressure and reduce the nitrates that create cell damage.
- Warfarin & other blood thinners are anticoagulants that slow the clotting process.

Sexual Dysfunction

Sexual dysfunction is when you have difficulty with any stage of the act of sex. It affects your desire to have intercourse and climax. Women can experience pain, making sex less desirable. Age, physical limitations, depression, anxiety, and neuropathy can also play a role in complicating this situation for both men and women.

For men, it shows up as erectile dysfunction, an inability to maintain an erection.

For women, it is a bit more complicated because often, there is more than a physical component to consider. There is also the emotional and even social aspect to this complication. However, research does show that when women experience a loss of sexual desire and vaginal lubrication, it is a result of their decreasing testosterone and estrogen hormones.

Blood Sugars

I recommend checking your blood sugar before having sex. It can be a vigorous workout. If your blood sugar is trending down, you will want to know if you need to treat it before you dim the lights, turn on the music, and light the candles.

For both men and women, take note that certain medications may affect your libido. Read the prescription information and side effects to medications you may be taking for anti-seizure, birth control, cholesterol, depression, heart disease, and selective serotonin reuptake inhibitors (SSRIs).

Smoking cigarettes may also contribute to sexual dysfunction as it impedes the blood flow to the vagina or penis, impacting arousal or sexual climax.

Female Sexual Dysfunction

The daily demands of life can stress you out or give you anxiety, inhibiting your ability to relax enough to enjoy sex. Or, being aroused may be impeded by a physical condition, such as having a painful bladder or yeast infection.

Sugar Happy

High blood sugar affects the nervous system, impacting the ability to feel and respond accordingly. Damaged nerves from neuropathy can also prevent genitalia stimulation, impeding arousal and limiting vaginal lubrication, making intercourse painful.

Menopausal symptoms – tender breasts, mood fluctuations, sleep deprivation, hot flashes, and the lack of vaginal lubrication — may also make intercourse painful, killing the romantic mood, and lessening the desire for sexual intercourse.

It is estimated that 40% of women experience female sexual dysfunction (FSD). However, women are less likely to seek advice from their healthcare providers on their condition. You do not have to suffer. If you are experiencing FSD, talk with your healthcare provider.

Treatments for Female Sexual Dysfunction

There are fewer treatment options for women experiencing FSD, raising concerns about gender health equality.

Medication

While there are a couple of medications currently being researched for use in women with FSD, the primary drug being prescribed is Addyi (flibanserin). The medication comes with a boxed warning from the FDA, alerting women not to combine alcohol with the medication. Prescribing healthcare professionals and pharmacists must complete an online course to prescribe this medication, which some believe has made it a deterrent as a treatment option for women.

Unlike Viagra that works immediately for men, women must take the Addyi prescription daily for four weeks. It peaks at eight weeks.

Hormonal Therapies

Androgen therapy, which includes testosterone, has mixed reviews. It is believed to benefit some women while having no impact on others.

Estrogen vaginal therapy promotes blood flow and lubrication. You insert either cream, a tablet, or a ring into your vagina. This may not be a long-term solution, it comes with an increased risk of endometrial cancer. Make sure you weigh all the pros and cons of this or any other therapy.

Lubricants

Lubricants will offer relief from experiencing pain while having intercourse. The lubrication creates less friction, making sex more enjoyable.

Vibrators

Vibrators have been on the market for a while. They stimulate arousal and contribute to the release of your natural vaginal lubricant.

Other Devices

Clitoral therapy devices are small pumps with a tiny plastic cup that utilizes suction to stimulate blood flow to the clitoral area. It can help women reach orgasm, and it may prevent fibrosis from building up in arteries leading to the clitoris.

Male Sexual Dysfunction

Erectile dysfunction (ED) for men is, in part, a result of neuropathy where nerve damage has taken place. According to the National Institute of Diabetes and Digestive and Kidney Diseases, men with diabetes are two to three times more likely to have erectile dysfunction than men who do not. And among those men who do have it, the men with diabetes may experience the problem as much as 10 to 15 years earlier than men without diabetes. There is no need to live with this condition. Treatment is possible.

Treatments for Erectile Dysfunction

There are many treatments for ED, which range from medication to penile implants to vacuum pumps. Sometimes depression can impact your sex life. Seeking out a healthcare professional to treat your depression might be beneficial. A sex therapist may be another viable option.

Pills

Medications used in pill form that help direct blood flow to the penis include Viagra, Cialis, and Levitra. One concern with these medications is that they can lower your blood pressure dangerously by interacting with other medicines.

Penile Injections

Men who are unable to take medications in pill form may try penile injections with Alprostadil. This drug causes an erection with the possible side effect of having an erection all day.

Why Maintaining Normal Blood Sugars Is Important

MUSE

Medicated Urethral System for Erection is a pellet inserted into the urethra that produces an hour-long erection within minutes. Side effects, however, such as redness, burning, and minor bleeding can be unpalatable for some.

Surgical Implants

Surgical implants work in two ways:

1. Inflatable cylinders are implanted into the penis that can be pumped up with liquid to produce an erection.

2. A flexible prosthesis allows the wearer to shape the implant into the position of an erection, allowing for successful penetration.

Vacuum Pumps

Users place a plastic cylinder over their penis and pump the air out of it. The resulting drop in air pressure around the penis allows it to become engorged with blood: an erection. Pumps have a fairly high success rate — 75 percent among users — but the erections they produce don't last as long as erections produced by other treatments, and users have to be careful about subjecting their penises to prolonged low to non-existent air pressure.

Some of the vacuum pumps currently available on the market are Erec- TechTM B2000 Battery Operated Vacuum Erection Device, Encore Deluxe Manual Vacuum Erection Device, Owen Mumford

81

Sugar Happy

RapportTM vacuum therapy device, and the SomaTherapy-ED SOMAerectStf.

Sex Therapy

The stress of not being able to have sex with a partner while eagerly looking for a solution may contribute to the inability to achieve an erection. You might want to consider sex therapy individually or with your partner.

Depression

One study has shown when people with diabetes and depression are prescribed medication for their mental health disorder, they are better able to manage their blood sugars. This study was completed by researchers at Saint Louis University School of Medicine, who reviewed 1,400 electronic medical records for people with type 2 diabetes. Of the group studied, 225 people were being treated for depression, and 40 participants had received a depression diagnosis but were not taking medication for depression. Researchers found that about 51% of people who were being treated for their depression with medication had their blood sugar well under control. Conversely, only about 35% of the participants with depression that were not being treated with medication had blood sugars well under control.

Speak to your healthcare professional about depression. It can make a big difference in your diabetes self-management.

Diabulimia

Women and men with type 1 diabetes who skip taking their insulin to lose weight are evaluated by healthcare professionals as an at-risk patient who may have an eating disorder.

The National Eating Disorders organization reports a higher death rate among women who restricted their insulin. For those who lived, they still cut off 13 years from their life compared to women who did not have an eating disorder.

The irreversible complications that result from insulin omission affect your eyes, nerves, kidneys, heart, liver, and gastrointestinal tract.

My mother omitted her insulin. She did not have diabulimia. In her case, it was a matter of inconvenience. Going home to pick up her medication took away from her spontaneity. Unfortunately, she did suffer by going blind, living with painful neuropathy and cardiovascular disease.

Treatment for Diabulimia

The best road to recovery is to find a healthcare team that specializes in diabetes and eating disorders. Join an online support group that understands what you are going through. They can offer recommendations to health facilities or clinics that were able to help them.

NOTE: You can find online communities in Chapter 8.

Your Personal Take Away Notes To Remember

CHAPTER 5

HOW MEDICAL DEVICE
FEEDBACK IS BENEFICIAL

Before you can appreciate the medical devices that give you instant feedback, help you adjust and maintain good blood sugars through diet and medication, I want you to know the history of diabetes.

We cannot appreciate what we have unless we know how we got here.

Diabetes was diagnosed and given a name over 2,0000 years ago by a famous Greek physician, Aretaeus, who took note of his patients' symptoms. In his formal observation and analysis, this is how he described diabetes:

"For fluids do not remain in the body, but use the body only as a channel through which they may flow out. Life lasts only for a time, but not very long. For they urinate with pain and painful is the

emaciation. For no essential part of the drink is absorbed by the body while great masses of the flesh are liquefied into the urine."

Fortunately, we have come a long way since then with the discovery of insulin in 1921 by Canadian doctor Frederick Banting and his assistant, Charles Best. Together they brewed a medicinal insulin formula that first successfully helped dogs with diabetes to stay alive, later becoming a life- saving treatment for humans.

The 1930s was a turning point for diabetes discoveries. Roger Hinsworth made his landmark discovery in 1935, distinguishing "insulin sensitive" (type

I) and "insulin insensitive" (type II). His breakthrough was instrumental in differentiating the two types of diabetes treatments. New, innovative insulins followed, made from beef and pork, offering better glucose management for people living with diabetes. In 1952, the long-acting Lente insulin was formulated.

In the 1960s, the first urine glucose test strip was marketed. One of my customers from Sugar Happy Diabetes Supplies, Dorothy Frank, a person with type 1 since 1929, shared, "To test your blood sugars, there were this do-it-yourself urine kits. Blue meant there was no sugar present and orange meant you were positive."

What if you were a type 1 back then, using the urine blood glucose testing and getting an orange color result, meaning sugar is in your blood? The next step was to take insulin to bring it down. It seems simple, right? Not really. *Diabetes Health* board member

Sugar Happy

Dr. Nancy Bohannon describes: "The needles were enormous, they came with little pumice stones so that you could sharpen them. They often became dull developing barbs on the end. And in order to sterilize them, they had to be boiled for twenty minutes."

You can imagine the fanfare in 1961 when the medical company Becton- Dickinson (more commonly known as BD) changed the way people injected insulin. Instead of having to sharpen the needle and sterilize it by boiling it, BD introduced a less painful device requiring less preparation with the ease of use — the single-use syringe, a welcome device replacing a laborious process.

Sulfonylureas, an oral medication that stimulates the pancreas to produce more insulin, was first manufactured in 1952 for people living with type 2 diabetes. It offered better blood sugar control when managed with diet and exercise.

In 1969, the first blood glucose meter was introduced by Ames Diagnostics. Dr. Richard K. Bernstein, a renowned type 1 diabetes physician and a *Diabetes Health* Board member who was once ridiculed in the medical community for his novel low carbohydrate diet, describes his first Ames meter in his book, *Diabetes Type II, Including Type I*: "In October of 1969, I came across an advertisement for a new device to help emergency rooms distinguish between unconscious diabetics and unconscious drunks when the laboratories were closed at night. The instrument had a four-inch galvanometer with a jeweled bearing, weighed three pounds, and cost $650."

How Medical Device Feedback Is Beneficial

Today, people with diabetes are fortunate to choose from a plethora of blood glucose meter weighing ounces, fitting in the palm of their hands.

The 1970s brought a new insulin treatment — insulin pump therapy. The device was large and needed to be carried via a backpack. Linda Fredrickson, RN, former director of the Professional Education and Clinical Services at MiniMed, describes her experience: "My first pump in 1980 was an Auto- Syringe, which weighed 17 ounces and had blinking red lights. People nicknamed them the 'blue brick.'"

For people who experienced needle phobia, the 1979 launch of the Derma-ject, a needle-free insulin delivery device, gave people with diabetes great relief. It did not have the best design. It lacked pressure, creating a jolt when injecting. The newest designs offer lightweight, pressurized devices that fit a child's or an adult's needs.

Also, in 1979, another vital test was developed to get a more accurate blood sugar measurement — the A1c test.

The A1c — sometimes referred to as the Hemoglobin A1c, glycosylated hemoglobin, glycated Hemoglobin, or HbA1c — measures your average glucose over the past 60 to 90 days. Blood cells form and die within 90 days. The A1c test records the memory in the red blood cells, giving us an average reading that correlates with a percentage. This percentage is significant to know because if the number is too high, it provides an opportunity to make lifestyle adjustments to avoid diabetes complications.

Blood Glucose Meters and What's Normal Range

There are many different types of glucometers on the market. When choosing the right blood glucose meter, besides considering the cost, important factors to discuss with your healthcare provider are insurance coverage, ease of use, maintenance, information storage, and special features that might be unique to your needs. For example, one glucometer from Trividia, the TRUE METRIX GO, is a compact device that twists onto a vial of test strips that can be stored in a GoPak carrier, which also includes a mini lancing device. It can store up to 500 time-date results, has full download capacity, and requires a relatively small .05 microliter blood sample. This kit has everything you need and is easy to carry, fitting in most women's purses and men's jackets.

For the visually impaired, an audible glucometer that talks you through the process will be more helpful, making checking your blood sugars easier. The first audible blood glucose meter I saw back in 1990 was the size of a medium office printer. I kid you not. At best, this only allowed checking glucose at home.

For the tightly controlled person living with diabetes, a glucometer that integrates blood sugar data with their insulin pump or a continuous glucose meter is the ideal device. Checking your blood sugar 4–6 times a day, adjusting your diet and exercising will help prevent diabetes complications.

Blood glucose meters and strips have come down a lot in price in the last three decades, making testing more affordable regardless of your insurance benefits. There are many blood glucose meter manufacturers to choose from — Trividia, Ascensia, Omnis Health, Roche, Abbott, LifeScan Inc., and a few more.

When healthcare professionals sent their patients to Sugar Happy Diabetes Supplies, I always took my time to get to know them. I asked questions about their profession, inquiring if they played sports, if they attend formal parties, or traveled a lot. Their answers helped me select and demonstrate the types of blood glucose meters they might want to consider, given their daily lifestyle and habits.

Continuous Glucose Monitoring Systems

The concept is simple. Continuous Glucose Monitoring Systems (CGM) allow people with diabetes to discreetly monitor their blood sugar levels on a real-time basis via a small device, usually attached to their abdomen or arm. If the monitor indicates high blood glucose and you take insulin, a short-acting insulin medication is usually prescribed as a therapy for you, an injection is required to bring the high blood glucose level down. If the monitor indicates low blood glucose, you may want to consume quickly absorbed carbohydrates to bring your blood sugar levels back up. Follow your healthcare professional's advice when treating your blood sugar.

The most significant feature of the CGM is that it offers valuable information about which direction your blood sugar levels are heading. If it is trending up, you might give yourself more insulin.

Sugar Happy

Alternatively, if it is trending down, you may take less insulin. Your healthcare provider who recommended the CGM will instruct you on how to handle the high and low blood sugars.

Both type 1s and type 2s living with diabetes benefit from a CGM device. There are currently four Continuous Glucose Monitoring Systems on the market —Abbott's FreeStyle Libre, Dexcom's G6 CGM, Medtronic's MiniMed 670G, and Senseonic's Eversense one of a kind- 90-day implantable CGM.

The FDA has approved the Dexcom G6 to replace finger stick blood glucose checks for people that are two years of age and older while the FreeStyle Libre, has been approved to replace finger stick tests for people that are four years of age and older. Medtronic's CGM sensor needs to be replaced in six days. Dexcom's sensor is good for 10 days, and Abbott's Libre FreeStyle sensor has the most extended usage as you only need to change the sensor every 14 days.

Insulin Pumps

The insulin pump is a medical device that delivers insulin under the skin through a cannula (plastic tubing) over 24 hours. This method of insulin delivery is referred to as your basal insulin. The idea behind the basal insulin is that it will deliver background insulin all day long, preventing blood sugars from going too high and minimizing low blood sugars by dialing in just the right amount of insulin. Once you and your healthcare provider have figured out your basal insulin and have it programmed in your insulin pump, you then will need to learn how much insulin you should give yourself when having meals. This is referred to as bolusing. Working with your healthcare provider will also teach you how many units of insulin you should bolus to correct a high blood sugar.

Both type 1s and type 2s can achieve good blood sugar control when using an insulin pump. But, not everyone is a good insulin pump candidate. Ask your healthcare professional team, ideally an endocrinologist, if an insulin pump is the right medical device for you.

There are currently three insulin pump manufacturers — Tandem's t: slim X2 with Control-IQ technology- designed to help increase time in range (70-180 mg/dL) using the Dexcom G6 CGM values to predict glucose levels 30 minutes ahead and adjust insulin delivery accordingly, including the delivery of automatic correction boluses as needed. Insulet's Omnipod tubeless system does not require a cannula, and Medtronic's MiniMed 670G closed-loop system adjusts insulin requirements automatically.

Pens, Needles & Syringes

Insulin pens are pen-shaped injection devices that contain a disposable needle with an insulin reservoir or an insulin cartridge. The device typically holds enough insulin to self-administer several doses before the reservoir or cartridge is empty.

All insulin pens are approved for single-patient use. They are designed to be safe for one patient to use one pen multiple times with a new, fresh needle for each injection.

The pen tip and syringe manufacturers have been "shifting to the shortest" ever since Mayo Clinic Proceedings came out with updated insulin delivery recommendations in 2016.

In keeping with that trend, BD, Owen Mumford, and UltiCare all offer a 6mm, 31-gauge pen needle that is compatible with leading pen injection devices. They are covered by most insurance plans, including Medicare Part D.

Several studies in recent years have shown that the short needles can not only be used effectively by people of all sizes but also reduce the possibility of injecting into the muscle.

What you need to know is that the higher the number of the gauge, the thinner the needle. A 32-gauge needle is smaller than a 31-gauge needle.

Typically, injection pain has more to do with the width of a needle than its length. Thicker needles can deliver a larger dose more quickly. Other features to consider with a pen tip is the ease of use; some people find it easier to use a "click-on" pen tip needle, rather than one that must be screwed on.

Both Owen Mumford and UltiCare provide dual chambers, one storing a supply of fresh pen needles while the other serves as temporary storage for used needles. Besides avoiding the risk of contamination, using a new needle each time can reduce pain that may be caused by a dull needle.

The V-Go insulin patch hides a tiny needle inside a device that resembles an adhesive bandage and is worn on the arm, leg, or abdomen. Pressing a button activates the needle, which delivers a constant dose of rapid-acting insulin. There are no batteries or electronics involved? The V-Go patch can be worn in the shower, but it needs to be changed every 24 hours. It should not be used by those who require less than a 2-unit mealtime dose.

Smart Insulin Pens

New on the market is the Companion Medical InPen, the first FDA approved smart insulin pen. It is a smart insulin delivery pen with Bluetooth technology that tracks your insulin dosing and pairs with a diabetes management app. It tracks active insulin, displays it directly on your smartphone and sends dosing reminders.

Novo Nordisk has collaborated with Abbott in connecting their pre-filled insulin pens thorough the FreeStyle LibreLink app.

Your Personal Take Away Notes To Remember

CHAPTER 6

WHAT AFFECTS YOUR INABILITY TO MAINTAIN NORMAL BLOOD SUGARS

Managing your blood sugar requires being honest with yourself. Are you overwhelmed or depressed? Do you understand what you need to do? Alternatively, are you one who can make an instant change after your diagnosis?

My mother had many reasons why she was unable to maintain good blood sugar levels. The most important clue I missed was that she was depressed.

Studies have shown that people with diabetes who experience high blood sugar are more likely to suffer clinical depression or nonclinical depression symptoms, such as having trouble concentrating, fatigue, feelings of guilt, persistent feelings of sadness or emptiness, suicidal thoughts, making them more vulnerable to diabetes complications.

Even though I had a diabetes supply store and a diabetes radio show, I somehow missed a critical clue with my mother.

Feeling frustrated at her lack of self-care, I went up and down the emotional scale. I started with being the supportive daughter. My mother always liked to learn new things. So, I thought I would appeal to her logical side, believing this would be easy for her once I explained what she needed to do to manage her blood sugar to prevent diabetes complications. When this did not work, I tried scaring her, raising my voice, saying, "You are going to go blind from your diabetes! Is this what you want? You will not be able to read all the books you like or drive to the opera or walk to places." I was sure this would motivate her. I hit all the critical points in her life. Her drive to care for herself did not change.

At my breaking point, I put my logic aside and tried appealing to her emotionally. "Mom, I love you and am scared for you. I do not think you get how this will hurt you in the long run. They call diabetes a silent killer because the damage occurring inside is invisible. When it occurs, it might be too late for you." This tactic did not motivate her, either. What was I to do? I was emotionally exhausted trying to inspire her by scaring her into taking care of herself. In the end, I realized there was nothing I could do. My moment of reckoning came when I surrendered. Just like seeing someone close to a cliff, knowing they may fall, feeling helpless, I became depressed. I could not believe my mother did not care about her health as much as I did.

One day, Beverly, a wonderful certified diabetes educator from San Francisco, invited my mother to join her diabetes class. After she attended the educational course, I asked my friend what she thought of my mother. Her response surprised me.

"Nadia, your mother is clinically depressed."

"How can you tell?" I responded.

"Just look at her body language," said Beverly.

I started reading up on depression and realized the certified diabetes educator was spot on. Her body behavior was classic to depression symptoms, and no matter how educated I thought I was, I missed this vital point.

The purpose of my mother's story is for you to first get a mental baseline of where you are in your diabetes self-management. This disease is not easy to manage because it relates to blood sugar management. Food and self-care play essential roles. Watching other people eat what you may want to eat is not always easy. For some, it does not mean the days of "I can eat whatever I want" is over. My former husband eats what he wants, checks his blood sugars before and after he eats, and injects more insulin if he needs it.

Some people with type 2 diabetes feel their diagnosis is a blessing in disguise. They lose weight, no longer take medication, and start exercising. For me, as a person with family members with type 1 and type 2 diabetes, I have learned to be more moderate. I am doing what I can to delay or prevent diabetes. However, there is no guarantee.

What I have learned from my family members living with diabetes is it is not about willpower. It is about surrender. Being perfect is impossible. Every day is a new day and a new beginning.

So, if yesterday did not work out, today is a new day. The most important thing is not to throw in the towel, but be patient with yourself. Change takes awareness and patience, and this can only happen with time.

Once you establish your mental baseline, then reaching and maintaining a good blood sugar range will be more achievable.

There are all sorts of factors that can make your blood sugar numbers vary. Do you exercise? Are you sick? Stressed out? Tired? Are you drinking enough fluids? What kind of diet do you follow, what portions are you eating at meals? Have you recently been to a lot of parties or social occasions where the food can spike your numbers? What medications are you on?

Once you know what shoots your blood sugar up, you can anticipate it by having a game plan on how to bring it down.

High Blood Sugar (Hyperglycemia)

The American Diabetes Association classifies blood sugar as high when glucose levels are above:

- 180 mg/dl one to two hours after you eat
- 130 mg/dl before you eat
- 100 mg/dl when fasting
- 140 mg/dl before you go to bed

It is crucial to track your post-prandial (after meal) numbers in two ways:

- How high they get after a meal
- How long it takes them to come down to the normal range.

These are the events that may increase your blood sugar levels:

Diet

Eating is such a big part of our social lives, at home, parties, dining out. When I started dating my former husband, I took him out to a sushi restaurant. He ordered fish on rice, seaweed salad with miso soup. It looked seemingly healthy. He checked his blood sugar after he ate and was surprised at how high his glucose was. Once he mentioned his high glucose test result, I remembered that Japanese restaurants put sugar in the sushi rice to make it sticky. After his dining earning experience, he limited the pieces of fish with rice and ordered Sashimi, slices of fish without the rice.

Sometimes when you think you are eating well, you may be consuming some form of sugar, which can be an ingredient in any dish you order. We do not usually think to ask if sugar is in our entree. If you check your blood sugar and it is higher than expected, then it may be a hidden or unknown ingredient that is the culprit. Checking your blood sugar gives you feedback so you can make the adjustment you need in order to correct an after-meal high blood sugar.

The Dawn Phenomenon

Nothing is more frustrating than waking up in the morning to a high blood sugar reading from your glucose meter. You took your medication, turned in for the night. So, what happened?

The human body releases extra glucose in the early morning just before waking up called the "dawn phenomenon." The increased glucose production provides energy in the morning to face the day. For people who do not have diabetes, the rise in blood glucose levels is easily controlled by the release of insulin. People living with type 1 and type 2 diabetes experience an increase in glucose levels that is not controlled by a release of insulin because either their pancreas does not make insulin or they are insulin resistant.

Medications

Prescriptions can also raise your blood sugar levels.

In 2009, the U.S. Department of Veterans Affairs conducted a study of 345,417 patients with and without diabetes, to see if taking a cholesterol-lowering medication increased their fasting plasma glucose. After a two-year period, they concluded that there was an increase in blood sugars for both groups.

Sugar Happy

Steroids prescribed as an anti-inflammatory for arthritis and asthma raised their blood sugar. Other medications that can increase blood sugar are diuretics for hypertension, antipsychotics, and anti-rejection drugs for people who have organ transplants. If you use birth control, this may also cause fluctuating blood sugars.

Sickness

When you start feeling sick, your body's immune system will fight the infection by releasing hormones and glucose. If you treat your illness with over-the-counter cold and flu medications, you need to be aware that some medications may have sugar in the ingredients. Make sure to read the labels first. Medications that numb your throat may also contain sugar.

Stress

There is no question that the American lifestyle is more stressful than people living in other countries. We have less time off, work longer, and get paid less. The American dream of a one-income family is not realistic for most. We are juggling a plethora of administrative tasks we need to take care of on a daily basis, like, keeping a schedule, going to work, buying groceries, paying bills, raising children, taking care of animals, family parties, and the list goes on. I feel stressed just reading my list. Add diabetes self-management to all your daily tasks, the stress tower may start looming behind you.

What Affects Your Inability To Maintain Normal Blood Sugars

We also experience good stress. Being excited about an event or completing something that was a goal can also raise your blood sugar. What happens when the adrenaline and cortisol hormones are released? It raises your blood sugar and blood pressure.

Women and Men Deal with Stress Differently

The American Psychological Association reports that women respond very differently than men when they are diagnosed with type 2 diabetes. Stressed-out women tend to turn to food for comfort, while men fight stress with alcohol and smoking.

How to Bring Down Your Blood Sugar

Sue Thom, RD, LD, CDE, former President of the American Association of Diabetes Educators (AADE), has some great tips on how to lower your blood sugar when it is over 200 mg/dl.

Call your doctor or diabetes nurse educator any time your blood sugar runs consistently higher than 250 mg/dl for more than two days. When a person with type 2 diabetes encounters a high blood sugar, the strategy used in bringing it down will vary from individual to individual. This is because of the differences in treatment concerning diet, exercise, and medication. It will also depend upon the guidelines for glucose control that you and your doctor have mutually agreed upon.

When high blood sugar does occur, some strategies can be employed to adjust the glucose levels back down to a normal range. These might include:

- Eating smaller portions at the next meal or eliminating a snack and eating foods with a lower glycemic index, then checking your glucose to see if it has made an impact.

- For persons with type 2 diabetes who have excessive weight, the loss of as little as 5% to 10% of total weight can dramatically improve blood glucose values, so just cutting calories moderately can achieve better blood glucose control.

- Lastly, choosing foods with a lower glycemic index, i.e., foods that do not raise blood sugar as quickly or dramatically, can help to bring blood glucose back into a healthy range. To test the glycemic effect of food on your system, you will need to do more frequent blood glucose monitoring. For example, you may want to compare the effect of brown rice versus a baked potato by eating equivalent carbohydrate amounts of these foods at dinner and comparing your blood glucose response two hours later. Some examples of foods with a low glycemic index are dried beans and lentils. The exact effect will vary from person to person.

Increasing Activity or Incorporating More Exercise

People with type 2 diabetes generally respond quite favorably to increased exercise with a lowered blood glucose value. A simple activity, such as walking 20 minutes or more per day, can effectively improve glucose tolerance and induce weight loss. Proper exercise can be effective enough to lower or eliminate the need for medication.

Increasing, Changing Medications, or Administering Them More Frequently

Although this is certainly an option, it makes more sense to address this problem of elevated blood glucose by implementing exercise and cutting back on food. These are measures that are less costly and have fewer side effects, but if they are not effective, a medication change may be indicated. If you are on the minimal dose of oral agents, your doctor might raise the dosage, split it into morning and evening doses, or change the dosing schedule.

This may also be true for those using insulin. Taking more shots per day does not mean your diabetes is worse. Increased doses may even bring more flexibility to your lifestyle. As a guideline, one unit of regular insulin should lower blood glucose by 30 mg/dl. If your blood sugar is 191 mg/dl before a meal, an extra three units of insulin may bring the glucose down about 100 mg/dl. It is important to note that this rule may change for people who exercise regularly (it will take less insulin to achieve the desired effect) or for those who become ill (they are more insulin resistant and may need more insulin to achieve the desired effect). The effectiveness of insulin is dramatically decreased also by high blood sugar levels. These are just guidelines, however. Remember to check with your healthcare provider first before making any adjustments to your diabetes management plan.

Relaxation Techniques and Behavioral Management

Relaxation exercises, including deep breathing and deep muscle relaxation, can reduce stress and help you deal more effectively with it. There are many apps available specifically designed to create images of healthiness. Behavioral management techniques also enhance the feeling of an overall sense of control of one's life and self-efficacy so that diabetes becomes a state of "wellness amid illness." When relaxed and in control, blood glucose values can improve.

Treating Identified Illness or Infections

Illness and infection cause a rise in adrenergic hormones, which increase the production of glucose in the body. This extra surge of glucose is part of the healing process but can upset glucose control. Thus, continuing to take medications despite poor appetite is vital. You may temporarily require more medication during periods of extended illness. Ask your healthcare provider for instructions on dealing with illness.

Monitoring on a More Frequent Basis or Monitoring Other Parameters

When blood glucose values exceed the target ranges established by you and your healthcare provider, monitoring should be done more frequently until the blood glucose returns to normal. This allows you to treat and adjust blood glucose as soon as possible rather than waiting until your next medical visit or next meal (which might be four or five hours later). It also tells you whether or not what you are doing is helping to bring the blood glucose down. Other parameters include ketone checks (done by urine dipstick via a finger stick to measure beta-hydroxybutyrate, an acid) if your blood sugar is over 250 mg/dl. Checking ketones hourly until they disappear is recommended.

Increasing Consumption of Fluids

Often, the inadequate hydration of some individuals will account for the concentration of sugar in the blood. All people (with diabetes or not) may want to drink 8-12 eight-ounce glasses of water per day. When glucose is elevated, drinking water helps to dilute it. Also, drinking fluids is filling, decreasing the possibility of overeating.

People with heart disease who take diuretics and those with renal (kidney) complications may need to be on restricted fluids. Check with your healthcare provider or dietician if you fall into these special categories.

To combat high blood sugar, the most important strategy is prevention. Prevention of elevated blood sugar is usually possible with frequent and consistent monitoring. If you have an awareness of your usual glucose response patterns to foods and exercise, it will be easier to plan out your day and prevent fluctuations in your blood sugar.

Low Blood Sugar and Nocturnal Hypoglycemia

What Is Considered a Low Blood Sugar Reading?

How do you know if you have low blood sugar? If you check your blood sugar and it reads 70 mg/dl or lower, you may need to treat your blood sugar. There are exceptions to this rule, and you need to work with your healthcare provider to understand when you should treat a hypoglycemic episode.

Low Blood Sugar Symptoms

Everyone can experience hypoglycemia differently. Some of the more common symptoms are: feeling irritable, confused, shaky, racing heart, argumentative, hungry, dizzy, loss of balance, and your sheets may be damp when you wake up in the middle of the night. At its worst, hypoglycemia could put you in an unconscious state, and you start to have a seizure.

A Reaction from Your Medication

Having low blood sugar can be very scary. Especially in the middle of the night when you are sound asleep, and you suddenly feel a racing heart, sweaty palms, and wake up from a damp bed. You may be shaking and feeling hijacked by your stress hormones.

I remember waking up in the middle of the night watching my former husband checked his blood sugar in bed to determine if the symptoms he was feeling needed to be treated before leaving the warm covers behind. Other times, I would see him standing in front of the refrigerator with the door wide open, anxiously reviewing his food options to bring up his blood sugars quickly. The first time I saw him do this, I thought it was a bit odd to wake up at 3 in the morning to have a snack. That is until I understood nocturnal hypoglycemia, a condition that usually affects people at night while sleeping.

False Hypoglycemia

My mother had an A1c of 10. She feared to have low blood sugar and sometimes believed she was having a hypoglycemic episode when, in fact, after checking with her glucose meter, her blood sugar was closer to the normal range. You may ask why did she feel like she had a low blood sugar? Well, she was so used to having her blood sugars hovering around 240 mg/dl that a normal blood sugar range gave her the false perception that she had a hypoglycemic episode. Going from 240 mg/dl to 140 mg/dl did not feel normal to her. It scared her.

I helped Juan, a friend of my daughter, check into the hospital for the same reason. Juan has type 1 diabetes. His A1c at the time was 17. He must have had a Guardian Angel watching over him. The only way he could bring his blood sugar down to the normal range without feeling panicked is by being admitted to the hospital. This was his physician's recommendation, and he was smart to follow it.

Juan called me from his hospital bed that evening, concerned about his blood sugar dropping. It was coming down from the 400 mg/dl range. Stressed, he was worried about becoming unconscious from a severe hypoglycemic episode. To ease his fears, I asked him to put me on speaker and call his nurse in. I introduced myself as a friend and advocate for Juan, explaining that he is used to his blood sugar being higher. I asked her to check his blood sugar so he would know where he stands. She did, the results showed he was in the mid-200 mg/dl range. This exercise did offer him relief. Rather than feeling like the nurse was not doing her job, it validated that she knew he was in a safe zone. He just needed the feedback to relax. I reminded him that was why he was admitted into the hospital, to bring his blood sugar down under medical supervision from the 400 mg/dL to the lower 200 range.

Spending the night at the hospital, bringing his blood sugar down, Juan left with a glucose meter, test strips, and learned to experience a new normal.

Glucose Meter

You need to check your blood sugar to ensure you are, in fact, having a hypoglycemic episode. Anything below 70 mg/dl is considered low blood sugar that may require treating.

Somogyi Effect

This is a process where your nighttime medication can lower your blood sugar when you are sleeping. Even if you do not feel the hypoglycemia symptoms, your liver releases glucose to fight the hypoglycemia (low blood sugar) by releasing sugar to bring up your glucose level.

Medication

Insulin and other drugs that stimulate the production of insulin may cause a nighttime low. Always check your blood sugar before going to bed. Remember to think about when your medication peaks to consider whether or not you should have a snack before bedtime.

Exercise

If you are exercising or exerting yourself more than usual, this can reduce your insulin requirements. My former husband experienced low blood sugar frequently after exercising. Once he made the connection between the exercise and his insulin dosing, he was able to achieve the right balance by reducing his insulin dose.

Diet

Are you eating late, less, or skipping meals? Taking the same amount of insulin and medication while omitting a meal, consuming less food, or not eating dinner at the scheduled time are other possible reasons why you may experience low blood sugar at night.

Preventing Nighttime Hypoglycemia

Check your blood sugar before going to bed to ensure it is within the range your healthcare provider recommends. If you have been taught how to do this or are a veteran of injection insulin, you may want to reduce your dosage as prescribed by your healthcare provider if your glucose level is lower than normal before turning in for the night.

Treating Mild Low Blood Sugar

There are many options for treating low blood sugar from your bedside. Some of the most popular and quickest ways to raise your blood sugar are by taking glucose tabs, glucose gels, and shots. These hypoglycemia options are available in a variety of flavors that allow you to treat low blood sugar without getting out of bed.

Some people put boxed fruit juice or pure sugar candy on the nightstand for an emergency.

The challenge in treating hypoglycemia is not to over-treat your low blood sugar, especially when you are feeling shaky, dizzy, or sweaty with a racing heart.

Glucagon Treatments for Severe Hypoglycemia

If you are unable to treat the low blood sugar yourself or have lost the physical sensations that alert you to low blood sugar, you should have a glucagon kit available. This is a prescription item. The person administering it needs to know how to use it.

When I owned my diabetes supply store, I met several people who, unfortunately, had hypoglycemia unawareness. Back then, the continuous glucose monitor was not available; emergency room visits for these type 1s were frequent and costly.

There are four prescription kits on the market today. Eli Lilly's Glucagon Kit and Novo Nordisk's Glucagon kit, both come with a syringe that needs to be filled with glucagon prior to injecting.

The Gvoke PFS is a pre-filled syringe ready to use for a severe hypoglycemia treatment. Their new Gvoke HypoPen single-use auto-injector will be available in July 2020.

What Affects Your Inability To Maintain Normal Blood Sugars

Eli Lilly latest launch in 2019 is BAQSIMI Nasal GLUCA-GON, a dry nasal powder that is delivered through the nose with no need to inhale. When it comes into contact with nasal membranes, BAQSIMI is absorbed instantly into the bloodstream. BAQSIMI is not recommended for people who experience weak adrenal glands or have glucagonoma or insulinoma. It can be taken if a user has nasal congestion or a cold.

Always ask your pharmacist about how to store and administer any one of these medications.

Accidentally Taking the Wrong Insulin

Sometimes people accidentally give themselves the wrong type of insulin. Instead of giving themselves the long-acting dose at night, they will administer a long-acting dose with the short-acting insulin, which could put them in a coma. The best thing to do if this happens is to call 911 to treat your upcoming hypoglycemia before your blood sugar becomes too low. The brain needs glucose to think. If you have severe low blood sugar, your ability to treat yourself may be impaired.

Hypoglycemia Devices

The continuous glucose monitoring system is one of the most popular devices for blood sugar management. The reason for its popularity is the built-in alarms that alert you to low or high blood sugar, allowing you to treat immediately.

Sugar Happy

The CGM gains more popularity every year as the medical device of choice for people living with diabetes, especially now since insurance and Medicare cover these devices.

The drive to be perfect in diabetes self-management is unrealistic. Accepting your good and bad days is part of your therapy. More importantly, acceptance is good for your mental health.

My mother graded her diabetes daily. She either got an A or F, a stark range that had no middle ground. Over time, this discouraged her from being able to achieve her A1c target. She did not check her blood sugars as often as she needed. She stopped taking some medication and she omitted her insulin. In the end, after having diabetes for only 13 years, she suffered all the complications.

My former Type 1 husband, on the other hand, makes taking care of his diabetes look easy. In part, his success is surrender. Getting a high blood sugar or having a bad day does not define him. He has 44 years of diabetes wisdom, knowing that the ups and downs are just part of everyday living. Thankfully, he has no diabetes complications.

Being Discouraged and Impatient

It's easy to get into a rut when you have diabetes. High or low blood sugar can be frustrating when your efforts do not yield the results you want. The question is how do you climb out of it?

My first piece of advice—don't be too hard on yourself. See your blood sugar numbers as feedback that you are fine-tuning and trying to figure out. Make it less personal by thinking of analogies that allow you to be more forgiving of yourself and allowing you to keep trying until you get to your desired A1c.

My Baby Analogy

When a baby tries to walk, she falls a lot. We do not watch her and judge her by saying, "Forget it. You will never walk. Why keep trying?"

Fortunately, the baby's desire to walk is not subject to a "good or bad" opinion of her efforts, which is why she will keep trying to get up until she can do it by herself.

As observers, we have the wisdom and trust that a baby's desire to walk will override their failing efforts. We do not look at a baby and say they are never going to get it. Why? Because we have enough empirical evidence knowing that all babies do walk, assuming they do not have an undiagnosed physical disability that prevents them from doing so.

Regarding your diabetes, remember, change does not happen overnight. The important thing is not to judge yourself, feel hopeless, or give up. Think of my baby analogy or some other metaphor that will help you be more patient and encourage you to keep trying different things until you find the right formula and success in achieving your desired average blood sugar range.

Your Personal Take Away Notes To Remember

CHAPTER 7

TOOLS TO HELP YOU ACHIEVE YOUR TARGET BLOOD SUGAR READINGS

The Diabetes Diet

This topic is perhaps one of the most significant issues when it comes to living with diabetes. In all my years in publishing, my writers and I have received more hate mail on this topic than any other subject we have covered.

Why? I believe when people write in, they genuinely believe that their diet is the best diet for everyone else, especially if they have been successful in losing weight and reaching their A1c target. With their best intentions, they write in to reprimand us for promoting what they perceive as an unhealthy diet.

When it comes to your blood sugar, what you eat does make a difference. Some people consume no more than 30 carbs a day, and some people eat 150 carbs a day. You probably are wondering, "Which diet is best for me?" The answer is, it depends on many factors. One thing I can tell you for sure is, too much sugar is not good for people with or without diabetes. Maybe if you were a professional athlete, eating sugar for endurance, this would be a different story. Even in this scenario, you must work with a healthcare provider to help you find the best balance between diet, blood sugar, and medication.

Some of the most popular diets work for some and not for others. Your healthcare provider might prescribe a diet that is specifically for low blood pressure or heart disease. Or they may prescribe a low carb diet to help you reach an agreed-upon A1c that is achievable.

Neal Barnard MD, an adjunct associate professor of medicine at the George Washington University School of Medicine says, "Plant-based diets work in a different way than 'conventional' diabetes diets. We now know that type 2 diabetes is caused by insulin resistance. Getting the animal fat and fats in general out of the diet helps repair insulin's ability to function."

Let's look at some of the diet options out there. Maybe you will find a more desirable diet that will help you maintain your targeted blood sugar level.

Atkins Diet

Dr. Robert Atkins, a cardiologist, introduced his low-carbohydrate diet in the 1960s. His avant-garde weight loss program promoted eating proteins and fats. Today, the Atkins diet has two low-carb plans with two stages: weight loss followed by a maintenance program. The Atkins 20 and the Atkins 40 carbohydrate programs provide a flexible meal plan where 12-15 of your net carbohydrates must come from vegetables. You also eat 3-4 servings of protein per day with 3 servings of healthy fats, such as olive oil and butter.

The one difference between the two plans is the Atkins 20 limits the selection of carbohydrate foods you consume while the Atkins 40 offers a broader menu selection, with 25 carbs derived from grains, nuts, and fruits.

DASH Diet

The Dietary Approaches to Stop Hypertension (DASH) diet is rich in fruits, vegetables, low-fat dairy products, nuts, seeds, and whole grains. It is moderately high in protein and low in total saturated fat. The combination has been found to reduce blood pressure in patients with hypertension.

Engine Diet

Rip Esselstyn, a former athlete turned firefighter, was concerned that most of his colleagues at the firehouse had high cholesterol because of their high meat consumption. He designed a 28-day diet plan that is plant-based for weight loss.

Flexitarian Diet

The name "Flexitarian" is a fusion of two words: vegetarian and flexible. This mostly plant-based diet is designed for weight loss.

The idea is to reduce your meat intake and consume mostly vegetarian dishes.

FAA —Food Addicts Anonymous

I knew four people who lived with 60 to 120 pounds of excess weight. They joined the FAA and experienced tremendous results. Their success in losing weight came from the support of their membership. The diet is strict, requiring that you measure protein, grains, vegetables, dairy, and fruit. No processed sugar or white flower is allowed. Their philosophy is considered a lifestyle choice rather than a diet.

Jenny Craig

This program is designed for people who want their food prepared with minimal effort. The benefit of the program is portion control and support. Every time you weigh in, you have the opportunity to meet with a person to discuss diet and exercise.

This is a fee-based program where you check in to be weighed and purchase your packaged food for the following week.

Low-Carbohydrate Ketogenic Diet

Many people with diabetes have achieved great blood sugar control with this diet. Because fewer carbohydrates require less insulin, the body dips into your fats, the stored lipids, to use as energy.

The American Diabetes Association recommends daily consumption of up to 130 to 160 grams of carbs, spread over three or more meals.*

Sugar Happy

Dr. Richard K. Bernstein, type 1, and a guru in the diabetes industry has been able to keep his blood glucose down to around 83 for years. He advises his patients to eat no more than 30 grams of carbohydrates daily.

Mayo Clinic Diet

The Mayo Clinic diet has two phases: lose it and live it. This plan offers quick weight loss followed by continued smaller, weekly weight loss. The goal is to rid you of your bad habits and diet saboteurs like eating out, watching television while eating, snacking on unhealthy foods, eating sugar, and too much meat.

The program encourages exercise and eating a good breakfast, lots of vegetables, grains, fruits, and healthy fats.

Mediterranean Diet

The name comes from the region where the diet is rich in fruits, vegetables, legumes, fish, olive oil, nuts, and wine. Red meat is not eaten often. Studies have shown this diet to be heart-healthy and a good weight loss diet.

Dr. Dario Giugliano, a professor of endocrinology and metabolic diseases at the Second University of Naples in Italy, conducted a study over four years with 215 people with newly diagnosed type 2 diabetes. The group was split into two. One was put on a low-fat diet and the other on the Mediterranean diet. By the end of the study, the number of people who required diabetes medications was 26 percent less in the Mediterranean group than in the low- fat group.

Tools To Help You Achieve Your Target Blood Sugar Readings

Ornish Heart-Healthy Diet

Dr. Dean Ornish came into the spotlight after researching heart health and stress from the 1970s to the 1990s. He is recognized for his revolutionary, no surgical method for reversing heart disease, which is reimbursable by health insurance.

His then unconventional technique included dietary changes, yoga, meditation, exercise, smoking cessation, and group support. The four principles are: managing your diet by making healthy choices with plant-based foods, managing your stress, implementing exercise and yoga, and experiencing more love with friends and family. He has 35 years of scientific data that proves his methodology reverses heart disease.

You can purchase one of Dean Ornish's heart health books or attend his fee-based programs.

Paleo Diet

Loren Cordain, Ph.D., is the founder of the Paleo Diet, creating a movement going back to the Stone Age where the cave man's diet consisted of whole foods, fresh meats, grains, fruits and vegetables, nuts, and natural oils.

Vegan Diet

This rich, plant-based diet excludes all animal products. There are two types of dietary vegans: the first is "strict" where there is no consumption of animal by-products, and the second consumes dairy and eggs.

Sugar Happy

Dr. Barnard's article in the journal *Diabetes Care* found that a low-fat, vegan diet led to lower A1c levels, lower weight, and better glycemic control.

Volumetrics Diet

Barbara Rolls, from The University of Pennsylvania and author of *The Volumetrics Diet*, provides a guide on the energy density of food. The theory is that very low-density foods, such as fruits and vegetables, will keep you full while high-density foods, such as cookies and potato chips, should be kept to a minimum.

She considers her book to be a lifestyle choice rather than a diet. The food plan consists of lean meats, low-fat dairies, vegetables, fruits, and whole grains.

WW (Weight Watchers)

Weight Watchers has shifted its attention from calorie counting to a point system. The point system replaces calorie counting by equating foods with a certain number of points. Each point represents 50 calories. You have the freedom to choose what to eat, but you have to stay within your points. If you exercise, then you can increase your points by the amount of energy you have exerted. The program focuses its members on losing two pounds per week.

You attend a weekly meeting or, at the very least, must weigh in. It is a fee-based program that offers group support and many recipes to help you stay on track.

Supplements

The Food and Drug Administration (FDA) regulates vitamins and supplements because they are considered nutritional items. However, the claims on the bottles are not always accurate. Some vitamins and minerals have science-based research to support their claim. Others do not. Even worse, some supplements put your kidneys and liver at risk.

A Cautionary Tale for People Living with Diabetes

The U.S. Department of Health and Human Services reports that weight loss and immune system supplements are marketed using unsubstantiated claims as to their effectiveness, lacking any research to support their claims. Almost 16 percent of the 172-weight loss and immune supplements purchased by investigators said they cure diabetes, cancer, HIV, and AIDS. Additionally, all vitamins and minerals need to follow the FDA guidelines stating that the FDA has not approved their language. Seven percent of the cure supplements did not follow the labeling requirements.

The scientific evidence supporting the use of supplements to manage diabetes is lacking in research. However, there is science-based research that validates the benefits of supplements to our overall health. A vitamin-deficient diet may cause disease.

It is important to note that supplements may have drug inter-actions with your medication. The recommended dosage for supplements varies according to your unique profile. Be sure to speak to your healthcare provider before you add a supplement to your diet.

Sugar Happy

The most popular supplements are listed below, and some can be found in the foods you are already eating:

Alpha-Lipoic Acid

Alpha-Lipoic Acid fights against free radicals that are harmful to cellular health.

Foods rich in Alpha-Lipoic Acid are red meats, rice, brussels sprouts, broccoli, potatoes, tomatoes, beets, and carrots.

As a supplement, it can cause stomach problems when used in high doses.

Vitamin B12

B12 helps the nerves and blood cells metabolism stay healthy, and prevents megaloblastic anemia, a particular type of anemia that makes you feel lethargic.

Foods rich in Vitamin B12 are meats and dairy,

Vitamin C

Research shows Vitamin C keeps the heart, immune system, and eyes healthy. It is found in fruits and vegetables.

Foods rich in Vitamin C are bell peppers, broccoli, brussels sprouts, chili peppers, guava, kale, kiwis, lemons, spinach, strawberries, sweet yellow potatoes, and oranges.

Tools To Help You Achieve Your Target Blood Sugar Readings

Chromium Picolinate

There is some evidence that chromium picolinate helps people with type 2 diabetes, high cholesterol, and insulin sensitivity.

Foods rich in chromium picolinate include meats, vegetables, grains, and red wine.

Vitamin D

The NIH reports that most people have a vitamin D deficiency, especially people who have a chronic illness and who suffer from depression. You can get a daily dose from taking a supplement, sunlight, and food where synthesis occurs in the liver and then the kidneys.

When taking vitamin D, you need calcium for absorption. It is a good preventive supplement for mature adults who are at risk for osteoporosis.

However, more is not better. Massive consumption of vitamin D can affect your kidneys. The Mayo Clinic reports taking 60,000 units a day for 60 days can create Vitamin D toxicity.

Foods rich in Vitamin D are cow's milk, almond milk, salmon, tuna, eggs yolks, orange juice, and fortified soy yogurt with vitamin D.

Vitamin E

Vitamin E is an antioxidant and guards your cells against being damaged by free radicals, which can make you vulnerable to cancer and heart disease.

Sugar Happy

It is found in nuts, vegetables, and fruits. But be careful. Research shows taking large quantities of vitamin E daily may increase the likelihood of developing prostate cancer.

Foods rich in Vitamin E are kale, spinach, broccoli, leafy greens, nuts, some seeds. Some oils are richer in Vitamin E than others.

Folic Acid

Folic acid is essential to childbearing women. A deficiency is associated with childbirth defects.

For children on the autism disorder spectrum, folic acid could provide an improvement in their communication.

Foods rich in folic acid are grains, citrus fruits, and leafy green vegetables.

Gamma-Linolenic Acid (Evening Primrose and Borage oils)

Although this supplement is touted to help an array of ailments, Berkeley Wellness reports that no scientific research reports demonstrate the benefit of taking this supplement. In fact, if anything, it can hurt your kidneys.

Foods rich in Gamma-Linolenic Acid are evening primrose, borage oil,Spirulina and hemp oil.

Magnesium

Magnesium plays a vital role in our nerves, physiological functions, heart, and vascular health.

Foods rich in magnesium are legumes, leafy green vegetables, nuts, and grains. Side effects are stomach pain and loose stools. Too much magnesium can kill you.

Melatonin

Melatonin is found to be useful as a sleep aid in normal healthy adults. It also appears that it may protect age-related macular degeneration by limiting the light that can create oxidative damage to the retina.

Foods rich in Magnesium are grains, fruits, and vegetables.

Omega-3 Fatty Acids (Fish and Flaxseed oils)

Omega-3 Fatty Acids supplements support cell growth, clotting of the blood, brain function, digestion, and muscle activity. It must come from the food we eat as our body cannot make it.

There is minimal evidence supporting Omega-3 Fatty Acids supplements. Eating foods with Omega-3 fatty acids has moderate research supporting its benefits. Fish rich in Omega- 3 Fatty Acids are nonetheless recommended for heart health.

Foods rich in Omega-3 Fatty Acids are walnuts, salmon, cod liver, and Atlantic mackerel.

Some side effects are loose stools and digestion issues.

Probiotics

Probiotics are usually prescribed after taking an antibiotic. Probiotics flood your stomach with healthy bacteria to fight disease.

Sugar Happy

The science behind it is still limited, and it is not intended to be an alternative to education or disease management.

Foods rich in probiotics are kefir, kimchi, sauerkraut, and tempeh, but the most common is yogurt. You can also take a supplement. If you choose a supplement, look for the research that supports the particular bacteria that is listed on the packaging.

Selenium

Selenium is vital to our metabolism, and it keeps cells healthy and protects against infection.

Foods rich in selenium are grains, cereals, meats, and dairy products.

The amount of selenium you need depends on your age and source of the selenium. Some soils are richer than others in selenium, so if you eat a vegetable, the composition of the selenium in the dirt will determine the quantity and quality.

Exercise

For people with diabetes, exercise is an especially good method to lower your blood sugar. It promotes heart health and weight management and fights against depression.

Before you start an exercise program, check in with your healthcare professional to ensure your new exercise program will be beneficial to your overall health.

Tools To Help You Achieve Your Target Blood Sugar Readings

People with and without diabetes face the same challenges in staying motivated to exercise regularly. Regardless of the benefits, how do you stay motivated? Find something that fits into your everyday life. Make it a lifestyle choice and not a task that you then have to stay motivated to do.

How Do You Get Started?

First, figure out what your story is. Why can't you exercise?

My story played over and over in my head like an old, vinyl record stuck on the same tune: "I am so busy running DiabetesHealth. com, I cannot possibly find time to go to the gym." After working long hours: "I am too tired to exercise today." I said this believing that tomorrow was going to be different.

One day, I got fed up with myself. My excuses did, in fact, start sounding like excuses. Once I realized that being too busy and tired was my story, I decided to take baby steps to change the way I thought and started looking for simple ways to incorporate exercise into my life.

I went into the shed at home and pulled my son's bicycle out of storage to ride short distances. Next, I found myself adding a basket to the bicycle so that I can go shopping. My bicycle now stays parked outside. If I can take my bike to run an errand, I will choose it over driving.

Sugar Happy

One Habit Builds on Another

Riding my bicycle strengthened my legs and gave me more stamina. I found myself calling my sister and other friends to see if they would like to go on a long bike ride.

Then a good friend I used to work out with on a regular basis gave me a three-month pass to her gym. All of a sudden, I got excited about going back to the gym. Not to exercise but to meet my friend, enjoying time with her at the gym, catching up on life.

I have another friend who asked me if I wanted to go on a hike. This friend walks three to five miles at a time. When she first asked me to join her, I was concerned I would hold her back. Then I caught myself telling a different story. I fought the "I cannot hike like she does" story and decided to join her, believing if she can do it, so can I.

Our walks turned out to be much fun. It gave us an opportunity to catch up on work, family, and our aspirations.

What Changed Me?

I no longer perceived exercise as something that will take me away from my responsibilities. It became a social event for me to enjoy myself, exercise, and catch up with my good friends.

Family and work will always dominate my day. Carving out time to work out with my friends is now one of my priorities. Plus, I have the added benefits of socializing and maintaining friendships that I value.

Tools To Help You Achieve Your Target Blood Sugar Readings

My tight clothes are looser. I am craving better foods to eat. My caffeine requirements have decreased to get through the day.

There is a domino effect to getting out of an exercise slump. I now look for friends who have a regular exercise program that I can join. This approach has prevented me from getting bored with my regime because my friends' routines offer me the variety I need to stay motivated.

Exercise Guidelines

Current fitness guidelines state that people with diabetes should work out for at least 150 minutes per week. This should include moderate or vigorous aerobic exercise, including running, brisk walking, swimming, and cycling. Resistance exercise, like flexibility training, is also recommended twice per week.

Hypoglycemia

Before starting your workout, check your blood sugars to see where you are. This is especially true if you take insulin. If you have eaten before you work out, don't assume you may not get a low blood sugar. Make sure to always have glucose tabs to bring up your blood sugar quickly if needed while you exercise. You do not want to feel shaky, confused, sweaty with a rapid heartbeat, or fatigued. If you experience any of these symptoms, stop and check your blood sugar immediately.

You are not going to make a better decision while your glucose levels keep dropping. The brain needs glucose to function. Your ability to make the right decision can decline as your glucose level goes down. Checking your glucose and having your glucose tablets will help you from getting a severe low blood sugar.

Learn your glucose-carbohydrate ratio by working with your healthcare provider, so you know how many carbohydrates you need to bring up your blood sugar while exercising. If you have a glucose tablet that is four carbohydrates per tablet, you need to know how many to eat to raise your blood sugar to the normal level.

My former husband used to experience hypoglycemia for two days after starting a new exercising program. The first time this happened, he knew as he continued his exercise program that for the next two days, he would be more insulin sensitive, thus making him vulnerable to a hypoglycemic event. He started taking less insulin and carried extra glucose tabs wherever he went.

Planning for a Low Blood Sugar Goes a Long Way

A 10-patient study that was published in *BMJ Open Diabetes Research and Care* provides helpful information for people with type 1 diabetes. When working out, suffering from exercise-induced hypoglycemia is always a concern.

Researchers found that by reducing the dosage of basal-bolus insulin and adopting a strategy for low-glycemic-index eating, patients can prevent exercise-induced hypoglycemia.

The strategy also appears to have no association with hyperglycemia or other adverse metabolic disturbances, showing that people with type 1 diabetes can exercise without worrying about the adverse consequences of hypoglycemia.

Hyperglycemia: Why Exercise Can Increase BG Levels

One of the most important recommendations healthcare professionals offer people with diabetes is to exercise to maintain good blood sugar levels.

So how can your blood sugar go up when you are following your healthcare provider's advice?

The amount of insulin in your system, whether from your pancreas or an external source, may be low to start with. Exercise may "burn" off blood sugar, but you may not have enough insulin, which is causing your system to burn fat. This can raise your blood sugar and, more dangerously, put you in a ketoacidosis state, a process where the blood lacks the sugar it needs and turns to the stored fat for energy.

Intense exercise, such as sports or weightlifting, can make the body release stress hormones forcing the liver to release more glucose. An insulin deficiency combined with exercise can stimulate the liver to secrete other hormones like cortisol and glucagon, which can raise your blood sugar.

Kris Berg, a professor in the Physical Ed. Dept. at The University of Nebraska, recommends checking your blood sugar before and after exercise. If your glucose reading is higher than 250, he suggests that you check for ketones and wait until your blood sugar is considerably lower than 250 before exercising.

To fine-tune your blood sugars when exercising, first, use a log to keep track of your blood sugar readings before and after exercise. If you take insulin, include how many units you took. Also, log the time and intensity of your exercise. Then make an appointment with your healthcare provider to discuss your findings. This way they can assist you in adjusting your medications and advise you as to how to achieve your desired blood sugar post-exercise.

The journal *Circulation* reports when it comes to protecting your heart and preventing heart failure, more exercise is crucial. While this may sound like common sense, a new study has suggested precisely how much more exercise we need. The current recommendation is 150 minutes of moderate exercise, 2–4 times per week. Researchers found that when people engaged in exercise 2-4 times a week, they reduced their heart failure risk by 20-35%.

How Exercise Can Affect Older Women Living with Diabetes

BMJ Open Diabetes Research & Care covered a study that examined how exercise affected older women living with type 2 diabetes. Researchers conducted a cross-sectional study using overweight women between the ages of 50 and 75 who did and did not have diabetes. They were then asked to complete low- to moderate-intensity exercises.

The results of this study showed that women with type 2 needed to exert greater effort to complete these activities. They also showed lower heart rate and higher lactate levels than the group of women without diabetes.

These measures suggest that when compared to women without diabetes, women living with type 2 diabetes find exercise to be more strenuous.

Family History of Diabetes Can Lead to Impaired
Exercise Response

The Journal of Applied Physiology reports that Swedish researchers have recently found that healthy individuals with a family history of type 2 diabetes have an impaired exercise response. Their study looked at 50 sedentary men ages 30–45 with and without a history of type 2 diabetes within a first-degree family member. It found over a seven-month period that the men with a family history of type 2 diabetes lost less weight than the men without the familial history of diabetes. It has previously been established that individuals with type 2 diabetes have a reduced exercise response, so it makes sense that men at high-risk will also have this impaired response.

Intense Exercise and Gastrointestinal Syndrome

A study by Monash University in Australia indicates that high-intensity exercise may lead to bowel damage. The study shows that blood flow is often redistributed to other areas, leaving the cells in the gut to become injured. Both the duration and intensity of exercise impacted the risk of impaired gut function and injury. This issue has been named exercise-induced gastrointestinal syndrome and has been the subject of some previous studies.

The Importance of Checking Your Blood Sugar

The reason why you want to check your blood sugar is to prevent diabetes complications. You now know what happens to the human body's organs when high glucose levels stay in your bloodstream. If you take insulin and don't check your blood sugar, then your daily diabetes self-management is a lethal guessing game. Why? For one, how much insulin you take for your meals will depend on your blood sugar reading. Is your blood sugar 100 mg/dl or 250 mg/dl? If you take insulin as prescribed but don't know beforehand if you have a high glucose reading, then the insulin you take may not be enough. Conversely, if your blood sugar is lower than normal and you take the prescribed dosage, you can experience a hypoglycemic event.

Checking your glucose gives you information. It gives you feedback on how your blood glucose responds to being sick, how stress hormones affect your blood sugar levels, how to avoid a hypoglycemic event when exercising, or when it is too dangerous to exercise.

You do not want to wait three months to take your A1c test only to find your average blood sugar reading will start compromising your health and your quality of life.

Tools To Help You Achieve Your Target Blood Sugar Readings

My mother's A1c was 10, which meant her average blood sugar reading was 240. She took insulin but did not check her blood sugar frequently enough. If she had, then she could have treated her high blood sugar with insulin to keep it hovering in a healthy range. For people who do not take insulin, they generally can cut back on their food intake and exercise to bring their blood sugar down.

If you walk away with one thing from reading my book, this should be it: check your blood sugar frequently. Although I do not have diabetes, I wanted my mother to check her blood sugar at least six times a day, before eating and 1 to 2 hours after a meal. This way, she could have adjusted her insulin and possibly delayed or prevented diabetes complications.

Checking your blood sugar used to be expensive and a factor in how many times people would check their glucose levels. In the 1990s, glucose strips were $35 for a box of 50 strips. Today, you can pick up the same quantity of strips for under $9.

Checking your blood sugar should not be optional. It is a commitment to your long-term health and to the people who love you.

If you get an A1c test and don't know what the number represents, the chart below will give you an idea of what your average blood sugar reading is.

Meeting with your healthcare provider and taking your A1c test four times a year will give you the feedback you need to make

Sugar Happy

adjustments to your diabetes self-management, keeping you on track to do your personal best.

Know Your A1c

Your A1c result corresponds with your average blood sugar. The percent stated as a number from your lab results tell you what your average blood level has been for the last 90 days.

Percent	Average Blood Sugar Reading
4 Percent	68 mg/dl
5 Percent	97 mg/dl
6 Percent	126 mg/dl
7 Percent	154 mg/dl
8 Percent	183 mg/dl
9 Percent	212 mg/dl
10 Percent	240 mg/dl
11 Percent	269 mg/dl
12 Percent	298 mg/dl
13 Percent	326 mg/dl
14 Percent	355 mg/dl
15 Percent	384 mg/dl
16 Percent	413 mg/dl
17 Percent	442 mg/dl

Inspiring Celebrities and Their A1c Stories

Over the years, I have had the pleasure of speaking to celebrities about their diabetes diagnosis and self-care. If you would like to read about more celebrities, you can go to diabeteshealth.com and type in "celebrity" in the search box.

The interviews below are of people living with type 2 and type 1 diabetes.

Actress S. Epatha Merkerson Brings Order to Her Diabetes

Award-winning S. Epatha Merkerson, television, film, and stage actress, brings a new order to her diabetes management: The *Get to Your Goals Program*, which encourages people with type 2 diabetes to know their A1c, set a goal, and take action.

Fifteen years ago, Merkerson was at a celebrity health event where good nutrition and exercise was demonstrated. A medical team was also present. They took her blood for a general health test. After the event ended, the medical team went up to her and said, "Your blood sugar is very high. You should probably make an appointment to see your doctor." When asked about her emotional reaction to her high blood sugar at the celebrity event, "I trusted it," she said. "I have seen it gone on unchecked. It was a big wake-up call for me."

Merkerson was diagnosed with type 2 diabetes at the age of 50. Forty pounds heavier after quitting smoking and not exercising, she was not surprised by her diagnosis. "I lost my father and grandmother to complications of type 2 diabetes," says Merkerson. "So, I learned firsthand how important it is to know your A1C and make a commitment to getting to your goal. That is why I am excited to work with Merck on *America's Diabetes Challenge* to help people learn about proper blood sugar management and inspire them to set and attain their own goals."

Merkerson's personal success in managing her diabetes comes with a support system. She has her "dining friends" who only allow her to order certain meals from the menu. They also make sure she checks her blood sugars. At home, her boyfriend helps by ensuring they eat healthy meals.

Her biggest challenge comes when traveling. In the past, she would skip meals and eat whatever was available. The exercise was not on her list. Now when she travels, she makes sure she has healthy foods to eat and goes to the gym at the hotel. At home in New York, she has traded the taxis and subway for her tennis shoes. She now walks as much as she can.

Traveling the country, speaking to people about diabetes, is a role she takes seriously. It is a grassroots movement where people can come together and talk about their diabetes at public events.

An Interview with Mike Golic

Mike Golic is the co-host of ESPN's wildly popular radio show, "Mike and Mike in the Morning." Before beginning work as a broadcaster in 1995, he played for nine years as a defensive tackle in the National Football League, including stints with the Houston Oilers, Philadelphia Eagles, and Miami Dolphins. About five years ago, he was diagnosed with type 2 diabetes. Since then, he has become involved in getting the word out about type 2, including the potential danger of hypoglycemia. He is a spokesman for "Blood Sugar Basics," a website and outreach program co-sponsored by Merck and the American College of Endocrinology.

I had the opportunity to speak to him about his diabetes.

Nadia: You are involved in a campaign to increase awareness of the danger of hypoglycemia among people with type 2 diabetes. It is a condition that type 2s do not worry about. Have you ever had severe hypoglycemia?

Mike: I am with you about how type 2s look at it. When I was diagnosed about five years ago, I was a little stunned because I was not showing any of the tell-tale signs. My father has type 2, so diabetes was always on my mental map, but when you think of type 2, you think of high blood sugar.

After going to my doctor and getting an introduction to diabetes, I came away with, "OK, you have this disease now, and what you need to do are diet and exercise." So, my athletic cap went back on, and I said to myself that I was going to lose weight. I stopped eating before I went to work out in the morning. That was mistake number one. The workout itself was very intense, almost like I was playing in a game. That was mistake number two. Put them together, and all of a sudden, I was getting the shakes and sweating, and my heart rate was going up. However, the athlete in me said to push through it as I would push through any workout where I was hurting a little. I told myself I would be fine. Well, I almost passed out. Luckily, I had some food in my bag, so I sat there and ate a little bit until everything came back.

After that, I talked to my doctor and asked, "What gives?" He told me that what I had experienced was hypoglycemia and that I had to be careful not only about when and what I eat, but also about the intensity of my workouts. He also said that I might have issues with the meds I was taking to lower my blood sugar. He said everybody is different when it comes to how he or she reacts to these things and that I would have to learn my set of reactions. There are many aspects to diabetes, and hypoglycemia was one I really didn't know about. I had to learn about it the hard way.

Nadia: Type 1s know the symptoms of hypoglycemia, regardless of how disoriented they are, they know they have to eat something. How did you, a type 2, know that you needed to eat something?

Mike: Well, I did not know at the time that it was low blood sugar. I was hungry because I had not eaten, and I felt horrible. So, I figured that taking a bite of something might settle my stomach and make me feel a little better. I did not know that that is precisely what I needed to do for the hypoglycemia until I went to my doctor and heard him explain it to me. I thought, "Wow, that is a heck of a way to find out!" Since then, it has been about educating myself about the different aspects of diabetes and how to deal with them.

Nadia: What's your routine now? What do you eat before you work out?

Mike: I am a morning oatmeal guy now. I love oatmeal and eat it every day. It gives me a good base. I usually eat that before I work out. If I work out in the afternoon, I will have a turkey, chicken, or a bagel. Whatever it is, I make sure there's something inside my stomach for fuel. It was dumb on my part not to be doing that before, since eating something before a workout is what you should be doing anyway.

Nadia: You are doing a quarterly A1c, right?

Mike: Yes. My A1c is 7.2%.

Nadia: Does your doctor want you to get that down?

Mike: Yes, he definitely wants me to get it down. However, I have made significant progress. When I would first get a sheet with all the figures showing the results of my blood work, I did not quite understand everything that was on there. Now I am at the point where I can look at the things that are highlighted, where my numbers are not in the range they should be, and figure out what I have to do. I only have a couple of things I need to work on — blood sugar and cholesterol. But I have another goal now, which is educating people about "Blood Sugar Basics," the Merck-sponsored program I am involved in. The website is www.bloodsugarbasics.com.

Sugar Happy

Nadia: Why are you involved with the program?

Mike: The website answers many questions and gives many tips about diabetes and how people develop it. Even though my father had diabetes, those were things I did not know until I developed type 2 myself. I have two football-playing sons who are large, and though they do not have diabetes, I want them to be educated about it and know where to go to find out about it.

Nadia: When you were diagnosed, were you overweight and not working out as much as you did before?

Mike: I was not working out at all. I had worked out so much through high school, college, and professional football that when I was done playing, I said, "That is it, I do not want to work out anymore." Although I was not working out, I was still eating as though I were still playing; not a good combination. So, yes, I was overweight. But even so, the possibility of getting diabetes was something I did not think about. I figured you had to be this 450-pound person who was frequently urinating and feeling tired all the time. I was not experiencing any of that. Yet, all of a sudden, my doctors were telling me I had diabetes. I realized that you could have it without all the tell-tale signs. That is why checkups are important, especially with us men. We do not think straight at times, so we do not want to go get our checkups. Men need to go find out what's going on.

Nadia: Men will not ask for directions or go to the doctor.

Mike: (Laughs.) That is exactly right. Thank God, women are not that way!

Nadia: But obviously, your attitude has changed. How do you view going to the doctor now?

Mike: I will make an analogy. The best relationship you can have with your doctor is like the one you have with a good coach. Every year before football season started, I was handed a playbook that I had to learn by heart, and before every game, [I was handed] a specific game plan. My coach made sure I understood all the plays and what was expected of me. "Blood Sugar Basics" is now my playbook, and my doctor is my coach. The comparison may sound simplistic, but my whole life has been football, which I have always treated a certain way. I have decided to treat diabetes with the same intensity.

Nadia: What's the best advice you have received about type 2 diabetes?

Mike: Don't leave the doctor's office until you understand everything. That is another guy problem, by the way. I would go to my doctor's office, and he would explain something in a way that I did not understand. Like a dummy, I'd just nod my head as though I understood it, then walk out of there. The advice to make sure you understand goes back to my game plan, where the doctor is my coach. I go to the "Blood Sugar Basics" website to find information and questions I can ask him. Instead of a one-way conversation where he is just telling me things, some of which I might not understand, I can talk to him about things that I have seen on the website and ask more pertinent questions. No more just sitting there and waiting for him to tell me things, or walking out and thinking two days later, "I should have asked him about this and that!"

Nadia: Do you think that most people believe that even though diabetes is almost an epidemic, they will be the lucky ones who will not get diagnosed?

Mike: Yes, the thinking is the same as when I used to be in a locker room and would see a guy who had blown out his knee or someone dragging himself in from a game after getting really pummeled. An athlete's favorite line of thought is, "It is not going to happen to me!" and the same thought process applies to diabetes. I knew my dad had it, but I never thought I would get it. Then I learned that it could happen to me. Getting people to understand that they should take steps against diabetes now and not wait until it is too late is important.

Back when my dad had diabetes, there was very little information you could get your hands on. Nowadays, you can access an incredible amount of information on the Internet with just the push of a finger. The "Blood Sugar Basics" website gives you the knowledge you need to work with your doctor and adequately take care of yourself. There's really no excuse anymore for not learning how to manage diabetes.

He is A Type 1 on TV and In Real Life

Forty-three-year-old stage and TV actor Stephen Wallem is a jack-of-all-trades when it comes to entertainment. Best known for his one-man musical revue, "Off the Wallem," he is also a playwright, composer, and director. Currently, he plays Thor, a gay nurse with type 1 diabetes, on the Showtime series *Nurse Jackie*.

Stephen was diagnosed with type 1 when he was ten years old. In June 2011, he teamed up with Novo Nordisk and the Entertainment Industries Council for a campaign called "Picture This: Diabetes" to increase awareness and encourage better management of the disease. A TV public service announcement featuring Wallem is currently being broadcast nationwide.

The actor recently took a break to speak to me about his diabetes.

Nadia: How hard is it to combine work on the set with managing your diabetes?

Stephen: Well, it is not like I work two hours straight, where I do not get any breaks. I am in a very fortunate situation where there's more downtime than there is work time when I am on the set. I have plenty of opportunities to check my blood sugar, and there's food everywhere, so there's no lack of something to eat if I need it.

Nadia: Has playing a character with diabetes made you more open about your condition?

Stephen: It certainly helps that they wrote in diabetes as part of my character, and that has forced me to be more honest with people

Sugar Happy

I work with. I did not use to do that at first, even in non-acting jobs where I was working as an office temp. I used to be embarrassed about telling people that I had this condition. I did not want to stick out, and I did not want to feel strange. But since the day I decided to be flat-out honest with people and not try to hide my medical bracelet, people, for the most part, have been completely supportive. If something came up and I felt my blood sugar drop, or if I needed an extra five minutes to take some glucose, or eat, or take my shots, boy, what freedom it was to be able to do it openly!

A little bit of education helps people understand when you come up to them and say, "I need to handle something right now. Can you give me a few minutes?" Ten times out of ten, they are going to be understanding. That is exactly what it is like on the show. As I said, I am in a very easy situation. I have a dressing room where I can disappear for a few minutes to handle something, so I am in an ideal situation.

Nadia: Has your role as a nurse changed the way that you manage your diabetes?

Stephen: It certainly has changed my outlook on everything. I will never pretend to be the perfect diabetic. Being part of the picture in a campaign to help treat and cure diabetes is important to me. I can help other people with diabetes know that everybody has ups and down with the disease. I'm a kind of figurehead in the sense of being somebody who can stand up and say, "Look, I know you can see me play somebody who has some terrible times with diabetes on

Nurse Jackie, but you should know that in my real life I have days when I'm right on target, and other days when I get frustrated and want to throw in the towel, and I'm in denial, and I eat terribly. Moreover, I pay for it later because my blood sugar is all over the place."

Nadia: It is great to be able to tell people that your experiences may be a lot like theirs. But isn't there a lot of pressure on you to be a perfect example?

Stephen: I do not feel any negative pressure. Instead, I feel a brand-new reason to treat myself better, not because I am being held accountable for it, but because if I can help somebody else by the example I set, I am also going to be helping myself. I really welcome the chance to talk to other people with diabetes. It is a very isolated feeling to have the disease. Although 25 million people are dealing with it, it is amazing how isolated we still feel.

I am so grateful to be a part of Novo Nordisk's outreach because being a spokesperson has benefited me as well as the people I am reaching out to. I have welcomed the chance to be an honest spokesman whose progress people can follow. I have committed to be open about my own struggles and talk about them publicly. Doing that helps others, and it helps me.

Nadia: Everyone has a different perspective on how people with diabetes should manage his or her disease. Do you run into different opinions about your own situation, and has that affected the choices you make?

Sugar Happy

Stephen: (laughs) I was told that at a conference in Washington, DC, that there might be people with conflicting agendas and conflicting statements. But I did not see that. Instead, I saw a room of diabetes educators and health professionals working toward a common goal. I remember meeting a doctor from Novo Nordisk. When I mentioned that after moving to New York, I felt a little lost and wasn't happy with my doctor, she immediately gave me a contact in Queens with one of the top diabetes specialists in the country and said she would call him on my behalf.

I walked out of there not only with a possible new doctor but also with a pile of business cards and website addresses. These were contacts and leads that would have taken me a very long time to research if I had started from scratch. So, I felt inspired. It was great, like a fresh start.

That is not to say that I do not still have my bad days. Diabetes is something you have to be conscious of 24 hours a day. You can never really forget about being aware of where your blood sugars are, what you should eat, when you should eat, and how much insulin you just took. I am on two types of insulin —regular insulin during the day and 24-hour long-lasting insulin at night. I check my blood sugar at least four or five times a day. Food and exercise are still issues I struggle with.

Nadia: Diabetes certainly compounds the problems involved in taking care of your health. Is that something you are open about in your outreach?

Tools To Help You Achieve Your Target Blood Sugar Readings

Stephen: Yes, and I will tell you why. I had a wonderful doctor in Chicago, who I went to see when I was in one of the "starts over" phases where you are trying to get back on track. I knew he was going to check my A1C, so I warned him that it was going to be very high. I guess I was trying to soften the lecture I was expecting from him. He smiled at me and said, "You know, all of my diabetic patients really struggle with this. There's nothing wrong with you for going through frustrating times." What a relief it was to hear that. I'd never really heard that before. Since being diagnosed with diabetes at age 10, most of the messages I had seen or heard in the media and advertising always tried to put a positive spin on things. I understand that, but it did not help me on my bad days when I sometimes felt I was the only one feeling that bad.

I think there needs to be a balance where more people are looking into a camera and letting other people with diabetes know that, "Hey, everybody has terrible times and frustrating times, and the best thing we can do is not kick ourselves for a misstep." We are in a really exciting time where we can talk openly about things we never used to talk about. People are open to the realities of other people's struggles.

Nadia: Have you had problems with your eyes as a complication of diabetes?

Stephen: About ten years ago, I developed diabetic retinopathy. I received laser treatments on both eyes, but, unfortunately, the bleeding got so bad that I needed surgery on both of them. I had

155

two vitrectomies on my left eye and one on my right eye. I had a wonderful retinologist in Chicago who did the surgeries at Northwestern. We were able to save the eyesight in my right eye, but the left eye was too far gone, so I did lose sight in it.

Luckily, I was put in touch with this great ophthalmologist near Chicago, June Nichols, who makes optical shells. She created a handmade shell for me that I have been using for more than ten years. It is essential for me to have it because I would not have been able to stay in the acting field with the way my regular eye was looking. Even though my left eye is still there, it is extremely smaller after the surgeries. The shell fits over my actual eye and moves with it. It is just godsend. You cannot tell which eye is bad, and even people I have known for a long time forget which one it is.

Nadia: What was it like for you and your family when you were first diagnosed?

Stephen: We still can't find anyone else in my family who has diabetes, so it is very strange. I stick out. None of us really had heard that much about diabetes when I was diagnosed in the late seventies as a 10-year-old. I had no idea what it meant when I suddenly started losing weight and urinating a lot. My parents took me to my regular doctor, and then he sent me to the hospital, where I was diagnosed. I spent a week there in orientation, learning how to give myself injections by practicing with an orange and a syringe.

Nadia: How did your parents take it?

Stephen: They did the best that they could, but they had so little information at that time. We had no real frame of reference. Nothing on TV or film even mentioned the condition, and there was nothing in the news about it, and we did not have the Internet. We had just what our doctors were going by, from what they knew back then. Obviously, today is a much better time for information. It is hard to be a kid or teen who's just been diagnosed with diabetes, but there's far more information and support out there now than there was when I was a kid. That makes it easier to handle.

Type 1 Diabetes: Manhattan Beach Teen Meets Nick Jonas

Rachel Humphrey, a Manhattan Beach, CA, teenager with type 1 diabetes, was granted her biggest wish (well, almost) when she came face to face with her hero, Nick Jonas of the Jonas Brothers. Rachel, 13, was selected to appear on the number-one new syndicated talk show, "The Doctors," but she had no idea that she would meet Nick Jonas on the set! The segment, titled "Giving is Good Medicine," aired on Friday, May 8th.

The plan began when the show's producers contacted the Diabetes Research Institute Foundation (DRIF), the organization that hosted the Carnival for a Cure event in New York City in 2007, where Nick first revealed he has type 1 diabetes. They were in search of a young girl with diabetes who is also a huge fan of the Jonas Brothers. Chosen for her outgoing personality and eagerness to be a positive role model for other kids with the disease, Rachel, who was excited about that opportunity in and of itself, planned to use the experience to spread the word to kids like her that "there is support out there and you are not alone."

While filming the segment, one of the show's expert co-hosts, Dr. Travis Stork, shocked her with the news that Nick Jonas heard her story and wanted to meet her. Feeling like the luckiest girl in the world, Rachel, along with her mother, Susan, was whisked away in a limo, emerging at a Hollywood studio where the Jonas Brothers were in the midst of a photo shoot. After Nick entered the room where she was anxiously waiting, they shook hands, sat down on a couch and began discussing their personal experiences about being diagnosed with the disease and its day-to-day management.

To her delight, Nick gave Rachel a necklace inscribed with the words, "A Little Bit Longer and I Will Be Fine," which are the lyrics to a hit Jonas Brothers song. She put it around her neck immediately, knowing that it will serve as a constant reminder of their shared moment — and their hope for a cure. Rachel is looking forward to watching her television debut and is crossing her fingers that other kids with diabetes will be just as inspired by Nick's message as she was.

"I could relate to him so easily," Rachel said after spending 10 minutes engrossed in conversation with her idol. "He has three brothers, and I have three sisters, so we both have a strong support network. Yet, we, even Nick, still get down sometimes."

158

Tools To Help You Achieve Your Target Blood Sugar Readings

A girl who loves playing softball and going to the beach, Rachel felt like diabetes had put her life on hold after her diagnosis on January 30, 2007, at age

11. That was just a few months before Nick made his own announcement in March. Rachel remembers her friends shrieking in disbelief. "He is going through the same thing you are!" Before that, the 13-year-old had been a fan of the Jonas Brothers, but when she realized Nick was working so hard to advocate for the cause they now shared, he became her role model.

"I went into the show just wanting to help educate others about type 1 diabetes, and I came out meeting a superstar," Rachel said, gushing about her experience filming the segment. "Hopefully, with his popularity, we can spread awareness and bring in enough donations to help researchers find a cure."

Your Personal Take Away Notes To Remember

CHAPTER 8

UNDERSTANDING THE PSYCHOSOCIAL ASPECT OF DIABETES

Family & Friends

It is essential to build a support system for yourself. My mother, brother, aunt, and former husband had me for their moral support. I understood what they

were going through and learned how to help them without judging them. If I had concerns about their diabetes, I would ask my medical friends for advice on what to do. There is a balance between caring and not stifling the family member who has diabetes. My former husband was able to tell me when he needed my help. My mother started having a discussion with me much later on, once she became more diabetes literate. If you are in a partnership and have diabetes, know that the people who love you also worry about you.

Understanding The Psychosocial Aspect Of Diabetes

I had the spouse of a person with type 1 write in to ask me if he should be concerned about his wife. He made a good observation and reached out to me for advice as a family member of someone with diabetes:

My Wife is a Type 1 Who Skips Taking Her Insulin

Dear Nadia,

My wife has been a type 1 diabetic for 20 years, and I worry about her because she does not always take her insulin. She is trim and seems fine, but how can it be OK to skip taking your insulin?

Below is a caring parent who is not diabetes literate and does not know what to do with her daughter's hypoglycemia episodes:

I Stopped Giving My Daughter Insulin and Was Reported to Children's Services.

Dear Nadia,

Help!!

My 10yr old daughter is a type 1 diabetic who was diagnosed at 2. This year she has suffered from severe hypoglycemic episodes to the point where I have stopped giving her insulin. The first time this happened in April, I begged the doctors to check everything…to see if there was some hormonal imbalance that could be causing this. They, in turn, accused me of purposely making my daughter sick and reported me to the state for child abuse.

163

Sugar Happy

Now, here I am again, and my daughter is back to having more low blood levels. Before it was just at night, now it is ALL day. Today her sugar has not been over 50 yet. She is eating protein bars, apples, carbs, juice...., and it is still dropping.

Sometimes family could be the source of your frustration, not understanding your challenges and making your diabetes self-management worse. You may have a partner who is not knowledgeable about diabetes and could make a request that could land you in the hospital. One woman wrote to me to ask for advice about her husband:

My Husband Wants Me to Ignore My Diabetes When on Vacation

Dear Nadia,

I have Type 2 Diabetes. I have been trying to manage things with diet and exercise. I was doing very well until we went on vacation and my husband ragged on me about it. He wanted me to indulge in the "good stuff" with him. I came away from three weeks of indulgence to feeling like hell. I am now trying to get back into my routine. I am hoping this is the start of a beautiful week and a journey to better health. Thank you for sharing your knowledge.

If you would like to read my answers to these questions, go to diabeteshealth.com and in the search box, type in "AskNadia," and the title of the question.

Whatever your needs are, they need to be communicated to your family. It is essential to teach them and your friends what you do know. If they do not have diabetes, they may not understand what diabetes self-management entails. Just like the husband who asked his wife to ignore her diabetes while they were on vacation. If he truly understood diabetes, he would have never made such a dangerous request.

Before I met my former type 1 husband, opened up a diabetes supply store, started a radio show, a magazine, TV interviews, and a diabetes website, I knew nothing about diabetes. Like my type 2 family, I did not know what I needed to know until much later. Luckily, my experience with my former husband and my work with the diabetes community for the last 30 years has taught me what is important when it comes to managing. As a result, I can speak from experience and can relate to both type 1s and type 2s. This is what motivates me to help you. Thanks to my family, in a backhanded way, they have taught me about taking care of myself.

Support Groups

My mother went to a support group and was surprised by what she learned about herself when the group leader, Lori Lorenzo, a certified diabetes educator, asked, "How did your family manage their health?" My mother had an epiphany; she started connecting how her mother managed her diabetes to how she is handling her diagnosis.

Sugar Happy

Grandmother Helen lived until she was 73. When we would visit her at the senior home, I always ran into her room first, excited to see her. Surprised by my sudden arrival, she would quickly start shoving candy wrappers underneath her mattress. The healthcare professional managed my grandmother's diabetes. Consequently, she lived longer than my mother. At the same time, the staff did not know that my grandmother spent money on the candy vending machines. If they had, maybe she would have lived longer.

Talk to your healthcare provider and ask them about local support groups that you can join. When I ran Sugar Happy Diabetes Supply, I went to the support groups to learn more about what people with type 1 and type 2 diabetes were feeling. I was grateful that they let me attend because I learned a lot about how other people manage their diabetes, giving me a broader spectrum than what I had learned from my family.

There is an organization called DiabetesSisters, where they help you meet up and start your own diabetes support group. I interviewed Founder, Brandy Barnes, a person with type 1, and asked her what her vision was for DiabetesSisters. "Our mission has remained the same since the day we started and always will: We are about bringing women together, whether online or in a central location, such as our conferences, or PODS (Part of DiabetesSisters) meet-ups, where women can support, educate, and empower one another. The three branches of our mission are support, education, and advocacy." Today they have added a session at their conference that includes a breakout group for family members. They, like their type 1 or type 2 loved ones, need support too.

Online Diabetes Communities

If you feel that your life is full, but you need support and don't have the time to attend a support group in person, online diabetes communities (ODC) are there for you. Everyone needs a place where he or she can connect to share their high moments and get support during his or her low points.

You can connect with me at asknadia@diabeteshealth.com. Every day, we post new articles on diabeteshealth.com.

- On Mondays, I post my *AskNadia* weekly column answering questions for people and families living with type 1 and type 2 diabetes.
- On Tuesdays, we have articles for people living with type 1 diabetes.
- On Wednesdays and Fridays, you can read or listen to diabetes research reports and podcasts.
- On Saturdays, we offer a weekly round of all the previous articles with links for easy access.
- On Sundays, we have an article by "Diabetes Dad" for parents with children with diabetes.

You can also sign up for our weekly e-newsletter or connect with me on TheDiabetesHealth Facebook page and Twitter.com/ DiabetesHealth. Most of the online support groups are started by people living with type 1 diabetes. Scott M. King, a visionary and co-founder of Diabetes Health, is a person with type 1 and the first blogger and person living with diabetes to start a medical supply business, radio show, magazine, and produce online videos. He began writing about his diabetes back in 1990. When the Internet became a platform for him, he not only wrote about his diabetes but invited many other people living with diabetes to come and join him. He provided an inclusive platform for writers turned bloggers, who credit their success to Scott's passion for creating a diabetes community. No other person living with type 1 diabetes has had this type of impact in the community. Scott's love for information has helped him fend off diabetes complications now for 44 years.

If you have type 1, Google online diabetes communities (ODC) to view your current options. If you cannot find a specific company, know that organizations can dissolve due to economics or get absorbed by another diabetes organization.

Some of the type 1 sites I recommend are:

- *DiabetesSisters,* which has a smaller type 2 audience compared to their type 1 audience, will direct you to the closest women's diabetes support groups or show you how to start your own group. You can find them at https:// diabetessisters.org/.
- The *Diabetes Research Institute* is an organization committed to finding a cure for people living with type 1 diabetes. You can view and support their work on https:// www.diabetesresearch. org/.

- *CR3* founder Charles Ray III, a type 1 who could not afford diabetes supplies, happened to resemble a famous TNT sports announcer. He was mistakenly identified as the legendary MBA player and acquired his diabetes supplies because of the mistake in his identity. His financial struggle led him to start an organization that helps people with diabetes who have limited resources to gain access to the medical supplies they need to avoid complications. You can access his site at www.cr3diabetes.org.

- Erin M. Akers is CEO and Founder of *Diabulimia Helpline* in Seattle, WA, a non-profit organization dedicated to education, support, and advocacy for people with diabetes who have eating disorders. The organization's website is located at www.diabulimiahelpline.org.

- Asha Brown is the founder *of We Are Diabetes*, an organization devoted to providing support for people with type 1 who struggle with an eating disorder. She is a member of both The ADA Woman and Diabetes Subcommittee, as well as Diabetes Advocates, and has devoted her life to spreading awareness of the deadly eating disorder diabulimia, which has become prevalent in the type 1 diabetes community. You can connect with her at www.wearediabetes.org

For Parents of Children with Diabetes

Pam and John Henry started an online program that helps parents stay informed about their children's blood sugars throughout the day. Their free online platform syncs the child's glucose readings for parents, schools, and healthcare professionals, allowing them to stay alert of possible life-threating glucose readings.

The organization's website is www.blueloop.myconnect.com.

Jeff Hitchcock, founder and editor of Children with Diabetes, started his site shortly after his eldest daughter was diagnosed with type 1 diabetes at 24 months. His vision was to create a platform that brings parents together online and at in-person conferences to build a community. I highly recommend his conferences for parents with type 1 children. It is one of my favorites to attend.

The organization's website is www.childrenwithdiabetes.com.

The *Diabetes Educational Camping Association (DECA)* is another gold mine for parents. They connect families with diabetes camps staffed by medical volunteers. Children who attend these camps can get away for weeks at a time without their parents and make new, lifelong friends. Instead of being the one kid at school with diabetes, they experience a camp where everyone is like them. Reach out to them at www.diabetescamps.org.

The ODC (online diabetes community) offers great support for type 1s, making it possible to make friends all over the country, helping each other stay positive and upbeat. The only downside is that there can be misinformation shared among community members. Before changing your healthcare provider-prescribed therapy, or implementing something you read online about how to manage your diabetes, consult with your healthcare team first.

Understanding The Psychosocial Aspect Of Diabetes

Not much is currently out there in terms of ODC for people living with type 2 diabetes. Since Scott's departure in 2008, some feel that diabeteshealth.com is now tailored more for the needs of people with type 2. The people who have said this to me are type 1 bloggers, and they are correct, in the sense that no one else interacts with type 2s the way I do online. However, my experience in living with a type 1 for 20 years and my lifelong experience with my type 2 family makes me unique in the diabetes community, allowing me to focus on both type 1 and type 2 diabetes information. Both are equally important to me.

Holiday Stress

Managing your diabetes can be very stressful, increasing the release of cortisol, a hormone that raises your blood sugar.

Molecular Psychiatry reports that when you consume high-fat and high- calorie diets while stressed, your body will burn fewer calories. Stress changes the way the body processes food, and the same result can occur with healthy fats.

A team of researchers from Ohio State University found that when women ate a breakfast that was high in calories and healthy fats after a stressful event, their bodies burned fewer calories. Plus, the women experienced increased levels of harmful health indicators within their blood. This included higher markers for arterial plaque buildup and inflammation – results that would be expected after eating a meal of "bad" fats. These findings show that stress can sabotage healthy behaviors that could lead to weight loss.

Sugar Happy

Attending Parties

People with diabetes face a more significant challenge when attending work, family, and friend parties. An extra treat or high-carbohydrate food could skyrocket a blood sugar reading to a critical point.

There is no shortage of criticism for people living with diabetes. You can be easily policed by well-intended people, assuming they know you have diabetes. If you are a fellow person with diabetes who finds yourself the designated critic of another person with diabetes, let it go. Until you walk in someone else's shoes, you have no idea how well they are doing under their personal circumstances.

Some Party Tips

If you have diabetes, don't judge yourself. Sometimes the stress of the event and the endless buffet of treats are hard to resist. If you find yourself giving in, check your blood sugars more often, and adjust your medication as you have been directed by your healthcare provider. If you can resist the treats and stay on a low-carbohydrate diet, "good on yah," as the Aussies say.

Respect other people's differences in how they manage their chronic disease. The operative word here is "their." You have no idea what you do not know about this person, and it is not always as simple as it seems. Not everyone manages his or her diabetes the same way.

When going to a party, remember to have a strategy. You need to be honest with yourself regarding how difficult it may be to resist all the goodies. I usually eat protein before I go to parties, making me full and less likely to indulge in carbohydrates.

If you are knowledgeable about diabetes, correct people when they make ignorant comments about the disease. Advocate for yourself. I know it is tiring listening to uninformed remarks about diabetes. Think of your correction as setting the ground for other people living with diabetes. If you educate one person, they will, in turn, teach another person. We want the domino momentum to build; the more people are informed, the less judgmental they will become about diabetes self-management.

Drinking Alcohol at Parties

Alcohol is such a big part of everyday relaxation and celebration for many people. From a hard day at work to sports events, birthdays, graduations, and weddings, not to mention the holidays, alcohol is as integrated into our lives as food.

People with diabetes can consume alcohol, but it depends on how well they can manage their diabetes and what type of medication they are taking.

Make sure you check in with your pharmacist and healthcare provider to ensure that any medication prescribed to you does not have a contraindication to alcohol consumption.

Sugar Happy

The most significant concern with drinking and diabetes is how your blood sugar responds. Several drinks will increase blood sugar. Alternatively, you may experience low blood sugar and become unaware of the symptoms because hypoglycemia can be similar to feeling inebriated — tired, dizzy, and disoriented.

Hypoglycemia

Consuming alcohol while taking insulin or type 2 medication can cause a hypoglycemic episode. It takes the liver two hours to metabolize one alcoholic drink. If you take a drug that stimulates your pancreas to produce more insulin, then you could experience low blood sugar. Too much insulin, in this case, may create a hypoglycemia episode.

It is essential to check your blood sugar before you go to bed. The recommended range is 100-140 mg/dl. If your blood sugar is lower than this range, the American Diabetes Association recommends having a snack.

Hyperglycemia

Drinking alcohol can increase your appetite causing you to eat more, making it more challenging to eat healthily. Extra carbs will raise blood sugars.

Other Tips

- Avoid mixed and sweetened drinks.

- Make sure you have eaten before drinking.

- Drink water in between drinks and sip your alcoholic beverages slowly.

- Never have more than one drink and wait until the alcohol is out of your system before you operate a vehicle.

- Wear a medical identification bracelet in case you have an emergency.

- Have glucose handy for a hypoglycemia treatment.

- Have insulin handy if you take insulin and know how to bring your blood sugar down.

When to Avoid Alcohol

- If you have a history of severe hypoglycemia

- If you have hypoglycemia unawareness

- If you have diabetic neuropathy

Who Should Not Drink

Underage adults, pregnant women, and people who take medications in which it is contradicted, should not drink alcohol. Discuss your prescription and over-the-counter medication with your healthcare provider to learn more about which drugs indicate no alcohol consumption.

Sugar Happy

Health.Gov recommends:

- 1 drink per day for women
- 2 drinks per day for men

Note: Not all alcoholic drinks are equal. The size of the glass, the type of alcohol, and the alcohol percent define what is considered one drink.

5 ounces of wine that is 12% proof is considered as one serving. The daily recommendation for men is not to exceed two 5-ounce portions of 12% alcohol. Using a measuring cup to learn what 5 ounces look like will help with portion control.

Let's say you want to have a beer while at a party. If you consume 12 ounces of beer that has 4.2% alcohol, this counts as one serving. What if you want to add a shot of distilled liquor? If you have 1.5 ounces of 80% proof alcohol, this will count as a second serving.

Ask your healthcare professional for their recommendations. Ensure you ask your pharmacist about mixing your medication with alcohol.

Alcoholic Drink-Equivalents of Select Beverages by Health.Gov

Drink Description	Drink-Equivalents
Beer, beer coolers, and malt beverages	
12 fl oz at 4.2% alcohol	0.8
12 fl oz at 5% alcohol (reference beverage)	1
16 fl oz at 5% alcohol	1.3
12 fl oz at 7% alcohol	1.4
12 fl oz at 9% alcohol	1.8
Wine	
5 fl oz at 12% alcohol (reference beverage)	1
9 fl oz at 12% alcohol	1.8
5 fl oz at 15% alcohol	1.3
5 fl oz at 17% alcohol	1.4

Drink Description	Drink-Equivalents
Distilled spirits	
1.5 fl oz 80 proof distilled spirits (40% alcohol) (reference beverage)	1
Mixed drink with more than 1.5 fl oz 80 proof distilled spirits (40% alcohol)	> 1d

Sugar Happy

One alcoholic drink-equivalent is defined as containing 14 grams (0.6 fl oz) of pure alcohol. The following are reference beverages that are one alcoholic drink-equivalent:

- 12 fluid ounces of regular beer (5% alcohol)
- 5 fluid ounces of wine (12% alcohol)
- 1.5 fluid ounces of 80-proof distilled spirits (40% alcohol).

Drink- equivalents are not intended to be served as a standard drink.

Too Much Alcohol

For women, excessive drinking is when you consume more than 4 alcoholic beverages per day or 8 or more alcoholic beverages per week.

For men, excessive drinking is 5 or more alcoholic beverages per day or 15 or more alcoholic beverages per week.

Binge Drinking

This is defined by how many drinks you have in two hours. What defines too much?

Women who drink 5 or more drinks within a two-hour period are classified as binge drinkers.

Men who consume 8 or more alcoholic beverages within a 2-hour period are also classified as binge drinkers.

Traveling and What You Need to Consider

Make a list. Traveling while diabetic is not always straightforward unless you take time to plan for your diabetes as well. Make sure to have a checklist as you are packing to ensure you do not forget any of your supplies.

Always bring backup. Whether you are traveling domestically or internationally, always bring a backup supply in case you lose or damage what you need for your maintenance and daily blood sugar checks. Have a copy of your prescriptions in case you need to get more supplies. If you are going to a humid place and take insulin, purchase a cool diabetes pack to ensure your insulin's potency is not diminished from the heat, which can make normal blood sugars challenging to achieve with the usual prescribed dosage.

Remember security checks. If you are traveling internationally, prepare for security checks. My former husband always packed his diabetes supplies in a separate carrier. He also informed the security that he had diabetes and wore an insulin pump. Less strict airports allowed him to take fluids in through security so he could treat a low blood sugar.

Prepare prescriptions. Learn which insulin options you have at your destination, just in case you are unfamiliar with the potency of the available insulins. Visit your healthcare provider before your departure to discuss your travel and to pick up an extra prescription to take with you. Photograph the prescription on your cell phone or email a copy to yourself in case you need it. I recommend doing this with all your travel documents as well. If you lose everything, you only need to access your phone or email to make copies of your prescription and documents. Also, buy travel health insurance. It is cheap for one year or less. Include the dental plan with the coverage.

Get assistance. Look up the International Association for Medical Assistance to Travelers at iamat.org or call them at (716) 754-4883 for information. They will connect you with reputable English-speaking doctors and pharmacists at your destination should you need them. If you end up having an emergency, you can also try the American consulate in the country you are visiting or local medical schools.

Check your blood sugar frequently. Different time zones can throw you off if you take insulin using a syringe or pen, so remember to check your blood sugar often. Your prescribed insulin dosage for night time might actually fall during the morning once you reach your intended destination. How you adjust the time zone should be discussed with your healthcare provider. For people using insulin pumps, like cellular phones, pumps have the added feature of being reprogrammable.

Study the cuisine. New countries have different foods, making counting carbs a guess. Go online and look for typical dishes from your destination. Print out the list of foods and look at the carbohydrates associated with the different entrees. Make digital copies of your research in case you lose or forget your list during your travels.

Be prepared when you travel. You will have more fun if an issue comes up with your supplies, making your back up kit, literally, a lifesaver.

Your Personal Take Away Notes To Remember

CHAPTER 9

OBSTACLES THAT MAY PREVENT YOU FROM ACHIEVING SUCCESS

Healthcare Costs

Few government data shows that surging prescription drug and medical costs are affecting the wallets of American consumers.

In August 2016, the cost of medical care in the U.S. rose by 1% – the quickest rate since 1984.

The cost of prescription drugs also rose by 1.3%, bringing the total price increase over the past year to 6.3%. This is the most significant year-over-year increase seen in the last two years.

Lawmakers and consumers alike have criticized these high drug prices, especially in the wake of the EpiPen controversy. The company raised prices so much that public uproar ensued, which forced the company to roll back the increases on the EpiPen.

Obstacles That May Prevent You From Achieving Success

A recent study has shown that the cost of insulin is continuing to skyrocket. From 2002-2004, the cost of insulin was $4.34 per millimeter, and by 2011- 2013, the cost of insulin in the United States had reached $12.92 per millimeter. A significant increase was also seen in per-patient insulin spending 231.48 to $736.09, and insulin spending was higher than all other diabetes drugs combined.

This analysis also indicated that the cost of popular oral diabetes drugs has either dropped in price or has not experienced a significant cost increase. For example, metformin fell from $1.24 per tablet in 2002 to $0.93 in 2013.

No relief is in sight for the prescription spending. IMS Health Holdings recently released data stating that U.S. spending on prescription medications will increase 22% over the next five years. By 2020, annual spending is expected to reach $400 billion. This number takes rebates and other discounts into consideration, and when using wholesale prices, spending could reach up to $640 billion.

Two types of drugs are leading the way regarding expenses. In 2015, cancer drug spending reached over $39 billion, while treatments for autoimmune diseases exceeded $30 billion. Additionally, the number of innovative medicines in research pipelines should ensure a variety of new drug launches in the next five years that will drive up costs.

The cost of diabetes jumped from $245 billion in 2012 to $327 billion in 2017. The average person with diabetes will spend 2.3 times more than their non-diabetic counterpart.

Sugar Happy

2020 offers good news to Colorado residents. Gov. Jared Polis signed a bill into law that caps the maximum copay for one month of insulin to $100, regardless of how many vials are prescribed.

Financial Resources to Help with the Cost of Medications

Once you are diagnosed with diabetes, you quickly come to share one bit of knowledge with everybody else who has it: the cost of managing it can add up surprisingly fast. There is an array of tools and supplies to contend with, including blood glucose meters, medications, insulin, and syringes.

For people who struggle to afford diabetes treatments and supplies, there is a way to cut down on expenses. Check competing suppliers for products that are being offered at a lower price point. For example, the Metrix glucose strips can be purchased online for as low as $9 for a box of 50 glucose strips. Their blood glucose meter can be purchased for $6.

Manufactures of medical devices and medication (pharmaceutical) companies have programs offering a discounted rate or no cost at all for people struggling with the cost of supplies. In most cases, you have to fill out an online questionnaire. This is how manufacturers can tell if you meet their criteria for free or reduced-cost supplies. Typical qualifications include low income and ineligibility for Medicare, VA, or specific government-funded plans.

Company programs may change over time without any announcements. Google any medical device and medication company by typing in the company name and the words "patient assistance" to learn more about their programs.

Here is a list of companies that are currently offering patient programs, helping you to reduce the cost of your diabetes supplies.

Glucose Meters

Free Test Strips

While there aren't any current programs available to get free test strips, some drug companies are offering discount programs to make these costs more affordable.

Abbott

Abbott is currently offering discounts on diabetes test strips through their FreeStyle Promise Program. To be eligible for the program, you'll need to have commercial health insurance or pay for your testing supplies out of pocket. Residents of certain states and those who use government-funded health insurance (including Medicare and Medicaid) are not eligible to participate.

Get Your FreeStyle Promise Program Card

You'll request your FreeStyle Promise Program card online, and for signing up, you will also receive a free glucose monitor. Then, you'll simply present the card with your prescription at any pharmacy

Sugar Happy

that sells FreeStyle products. The company has stated that you will play as low as $15 per prescription with the card, and this will typically get about a month's worth of test strips. However, savings will vary depending on the type of insurance you use and the number of strips that you purchase.

Roche

The Roche AccuChek Guide SimplePay Subscription Program ships test strips directly to your door or preferred pharmacy for a discount. In order to join the program, you cannot have medical or prescription medication coverage through any government program, including Medicare and Medicaid. You do not have to have healthcare insurance to be eligible.

Get Your Accu-Chek Preferred Savings Program

To get a card to start saving, go online to fill out a simple form. You can also receive it from a pharmacist that sells Accu-Chek products. Simply present the card with your prescription for your test strips every time that you go in for a refill. Since the card never expires, you'll be able to use it as long as you need to.

The program discounts the cost of test strips significantly. You can order anywhere from 50 strips for $19.99 to 300 strips for $69.99. You'll then receive regular shipments every one, two, three, or six months.

Organizations that Help with
Diabetes Supplies

Several healthcare organizations and drug companies are currently offering programs to help diabetics to better manage their disease with free or low-cost supplies.

Abbott

Abbott is currently offering discounts on diabetes test strips through their FreeStyle Promise Program. To be eligible for the program, you will need to have commercial health insurance or pay for your testing supplies out of pocket. People who use government-funded health insurance (including Medicare and Medicaid) are not eligible to participate. There may be further stipulations depending on what state you live in, so be sure to ask. To get your free Freestyle glucose meter, you will first need to complete a series of questions on the company's website. Once submitted and qualified, you can print your free Freestyle Promise Card. Next, visit your healthcare provider to get a prescription for Freestyle Lite test strips and take both documents into your local pharmacy. After you pick up your free glucose meter, you will pay as little as $15 for your test strips every time that you fill your prescription.

Roche

While Roche previously offered a Patient Assistance Program, this plan has been replaced with the current Accu-Chek Preferred savings Program. Once found eligible, you will pay the preferred

Sugar Happy

rate on Accu-Chek strips, even if your test strips aren't being covered by the pharmacy benefits of your health insurance.

Anyone with private health insurance is eligible, except Massachusetts residents. People with government health coverage (including Medicare or Medicaid) are not eligible, nor are people who pay out of pocket.

Free Test Strips

Abbott

(See description under Glucose Meters.)

Roche

(See description under Glucose Meters.)

Free Insulin Syringes

Should you need help paying for your syringes in order to administer your insulin, programs are available to help with the costs.

The BD Insulin Syringe Assist Program

BD is a medical technology organization that manufactures and sells a range of medical supplies, lab equipment, diagnostic products, and other devices. BD Medical has a Diabetes Care department that provides a variety of testing supplies, including syringes, pen needles, lancets, and disposal products.

About BD Insulin Syringes

BD Syringes are designed for single use and are labeled accordingly. The company is currently manufacturing U-100 insulin syringes that include Ultra-Fine needles in the following sizes:

- 1 mL (100 unit)
- 1/2 mL (50 unit)
- 3/10 mL (30 unit)
- 3/10 mL with half unit markings

There are also three available options for needle lengths: 12.7 mm, 8 mm, and 6 mm, although BD recommends using the 6 mm since research has shown that short needles tend to be safer and better tolerated than longer options. BDs syringes, pen needles, and accessories are available for purchase at most pharmacies, and they can also be received by mail from durable medical supply companies. If your pharmacy does not have the specific BD insulin syringe that you need, ask the pharmacist to order it by calling BD Customer Service.

Get Help Paying for Your Insulin Syringes

BD Medical's Diabetes Care division is currently offering a patient assistance program for diabetics who are using BD Ultra-Fine Insulin Syringes and cannot pay for them due to a lack of health insurance or low-income status. To qualify, you need to meet financial and other criteria, and you cannot have access to government sponsored insurance like Medicaid or Medicare.

Sugar Happy

To apply for this program, you will need to call the company directly at 1-888-367-8517, and you can visit their website for additional information about products. If it is found that you are eligible for the program, you will receive your 90-day supply of BD Ultra-Fine Insulin Syringes for a $15.00 copay.

Free Insulin

If you are having a hard time paying for your insulin, consider applying for a prescription assistance program to help with your costs.

Lilly Cares

Lilly Cares is a program that provides free Lilly medications to patients via their doctor's office. A variety of medications are available for coverage if certain eligibility criteria are met, but for diabetics, insulin medications like Humalog U100, Humalog U200, Humalog Mix 50/50, and Humalog Mix 75/25 will be of greatest interest.

Eligibility Requirements

To receive prescription assistance for insulin through the Lilly Cares program, you need to meet the following criteria:

- A permanent and legal resident of the United States
- Not enrolled in or eligible for Medicaid, full Low-Income Subsidy, or medical benefits from the Veteran's Administration

- Must have no prescription drug coverage or be enrolled in Medicare Part D
- If enrolled in Medicare Part D, applicants must have spent a minimum of $1,100 on prescription medication for the calendar year.
- Have a valid prescription for a drug available through the Lilly Cares program
- Meet income guidelines (ex. Maximum household income of $77,250 for a family of four)

Getting Your Medication

To apply, you'll need to download the application and complete it with your doctor. Once approved, you will receive up to a 120-day supply of your insulin shipped directly to your doctor's office. You will be eligible for prescription refills for your one-year enrollment period.

NovoLog Patient Assistance Program

The NovoLog Patient Assistance Program helps to make prescriptions affordable for people who may have trouble paying for them. The program is free for qualified individuals, and there is no monthly fee or registration charge for participating.

Eligibility Requirements

To receive prescription assistance for insulin through the NovoLog Patient Assistance Program you need to meet the following criteria:

Sugar Happy

- A permanent and legal resident of the United States
- Cannot be enrolled in a government-sponsored program, including Medicaid or Medicare. There are some exceptions, such as those on Medicare Part D who have spent over $1,000 on prescription medications in the past year and those who have been denied Medicaid.
- Not eligible for VA prescription drug benefits.
- Not enrolled in a private prescription drug program, including a PPO or HMO
- Meet income guidelines in which the total household income is at or below 400% of the U.S. federal poverty level

Sanofi Aventis

Sanofi Patient Connection offers help to make prescriptions affordable for people who may have trouble paying for them. The program is free for qualified individuals, and there is no monthly fee or registration charge for participating.

Eligibility Requirements:

To receive prescription assistance for insulin through the Sanofi Patient Connection, you need to meet the following criteria:

- Be a permanent and legal resident of the United States
- Work with a U.S. healthcare professional who is licensed to prescribe
- Must have no insurance prescription drug coverage

- Must not qualify for Medicare or Medicaid. Medicare Part D may offer eligibility
- Must meet income guidelines (ex. Maximum household income of $72,750 for a family of four)

Medication

Xubex

Xubex Pharmacy services offer affordable brand-named medications, and their Patient Assistance Program (PAP) works to help people who aren't able to pay for the high costs of their meds. Qualifying people without prescription drug coverage can receive free or low-cost medicines through the organization, and for people with diabetes, the most commonly sought-after medication available through the organization is metformin.

Novo Nordisk

The Novo Nordisk Patient Assistance Program (PAP) offers free diabetes medications to individuals who qualify. If approved, you can receive a free 120-day supply of your drugs, and they will be sent to your healthcare provider's office to be picked up at your convenience. Novo Nordisk then contacts your healthcare provider automatically 90 days later to approve a refill of the medication.

If you need assistance with paying for your diabetes medications, download an application and complete your portion. Then, you will need to obtain proof of your income before taking your application to your healthcare provider so that he/she can complete the "Health Care

Sugar Happy

Practitioner" portion. You will then send in your application for processing, and if you have additional questions, you can contact Customer service at 866-310-7549.

Pfizer

Pfizer RxPathways is an assistance program that provides eligible people with access to medicine at a reduced cost or for free. To apply, visit the website and enter your diabetes medications, such as Glucotrol, and then check your eligibility. Questions to determine if you are eligible include whether or not you have prescription coverage, the number of people in your household, and your total annual household income. You can then print an application to apply, or you can contact Customer Service at 1-866-706-2400 to determine if you qualify.

The Cure or Reversing Diabetes

Diabetes 101

Type 1 Diabetes

The cure for type 1 diabetes is a multi-billion-dollar question. There are no known cures. People with type 1 diabetes require insulin to live.

A few have achieved some success with organ transplants. After surgery, the organ transplant recipients no longer required insulin, and some consider themselves "cured," meaning insulin injections are not required.

Obstacles That May Prevent You From Achieving Success

Organ transplant recipients have to take anti-rejection medication to ensure their body does not attack the new organ. Unfortunately, some of these medications list diabetes as a side effect.

What is considered more revered for people living with type 1 diabetes is the artificial pancreas. The artificial pancreas combines medical devices with a predicting algorithm, a continuous glucose monitor, and an insulin pump system. If set on automatic, the system can look at your blood glucose patterns and adjust your insulin requirements accordingly.

For people living with type 1 diabetes, this is not a cure, but for some, it is considered the closest thing to a cure.

Type 2 Diabetes

There is no cure for type 2 diabetes. However, many people can maintain good blood sugar control with diet and exercise. If success is not achieved with diet and exercise, physicians will generally put you on medication to help achieve good blood sugar.

The medications can be oral, insulin, or another class of injectable medication. Your healthcare provider will determine the combination, if any, to maintain normal blood sugar levels.

What is the problem with the terms "curing" or "reversing" type 2 diabetes? They are marketing terms that play on people's vulnerability. It implies that your biochemistry reverses its insulin resistance permanently, meaning a person with diabetes suddenly becomes cured and does not have diabetes.

Sugar Happy

How Food Impacts Diabetes

Food raises blood sugars. Some foods like pasta, pizza, rice, and desserts raise your blood sugars a lot. Other foods such as lean proteins (e.g., fish, chicken) and fresh blueberries do not raise your blood sugars like pasta or pizza.

Eating foods that don't dramatically raise your blood sugar is good for your health. It also can keep your blood sugars in the normal range. Maintaining healthy blood sugar can often be achieved with diet and exercise.

People who don't have diabetes will not experience the same elevated blood sugars that a person with diabetes will. If a person with diabetes starts their morning with a large glass of orange juice and a bagel, then has two pieces of pizza for lunch with a soft drink and follows it with a large pasta dish for dinner and ice cream sundae for dessert, this could land them in the hospital, even if they are taking a supplement that promotes better blood sugars.

For someone without diabetes, they may not feel good after eating a high- carbohydrate meal. However, this would not land them in the hospital unless they contracted something from the food or preparation of the food, which made them ill enough to seek emergency care.

When we eat food, one of several hormones released in the body is insulin, a hormone that converts food into energy. Not enough insulin gives you high blood sugar, while too much insulin gives you low blood sugar.

Hindsight is 20/20

After my mother underwent vascular surgery, she was in the hospital for her recovery. I would visit her for long periods, and we would hang out and watch TV. Well, I watched it. She could only listen.

I remember asking her how she was feeling. Her answer surprised me. Her response was more rhetorical about how she managed her diabetes over 13 years. "You know, Nadia, I saw my mother manage her diabetes, and she seemed fine. I had no idea that high blood sugars can do this much damage. I wish I had managed my diabetes differently."

Hindsight is 20/20. If we could look into the future and feel the diabetes complications from high blood sugar, I believe most people would manage it differently. My question to you, and I ask this with no judgment, would you rather have short-term gratification by eating what you want, not taking medication, and not checking your blood sugar and ignoring your diabetes or long-terms benefits for doing what you can do to delay or prevent diabetes complications? It's your call.

You've Got This

If you have been feeling overwhelmed with your diabetes, now you know why.

Before your diagnosis, you may have had symptoms that scared you, such as blurry vision, unquenchable thirst, and going to the restroom frequently. Once you get your diagnosis, you are relieved that it has a name, but then you are in shock, scared, thinking of all the horrible things you have heard or seen on the television screen about diabetes.

Sitting in front of a healthcare professional, they teach you how to care for a chronic illness when you still have not wrapped your head around the diagnosis, and it seems like you are listening to a foreign language. They use terms like "your A1c target range" and "good blood sugar reading before and after a meal." To make things more complicated, they ask you to buy a medical device called a blood glucose meter, then they train you on how to use it. Feeling scared and apprehensive about lancing your finger to draw blood, you are not embracing the process. It is not intuitive. Not only that, you need to do it several times a day.

You start testing your blood sugar regularly as instructed. The readings from the glucose meter are all over the chart, you do not understand it. Even worse, you feel discouraged after checking your blood glucose, deciding it is best not to know because it upsets you, making you feel powerless.

Over time, you find checking regularly becomes less scary. You have practiced enough and feel confident about using your meter. In fact, you start looking at other medical devices, like a continuous glucose monitoring system that can help you see which way your blood sugar is trending, allowing you to as instructed by your healthcare provider.

Obstacles That May Prevent You From Achieving Success

Ordering your supplies is no longer confusing. Knowing how to manage your blood sugar with diet, exercise, and/or medication becomes natural. You've got this down. You are feeling good.

When I had my Sugar Happy Diabetes Supplies business, I remember speaking to a person with type 2 diabetes and asking him if he takes insulin. He said he did. I asked him what type of insulin therapy he was on. He said: "I do not know. It is a pill." Insulin is not distributed in a pill form. This gave me insight into how well he understood his medication.

Educating yourself on what you are taking and how it works is empowering.

People with type 1 have to take insulin. If they do not take insulin as prescribed, they can unintentionally find their way to the emergency room at the nearest hospital. For type 2s, taking medication in a pill form might give you the illusion, "this is all I have to do. I am not that bad," not realizing that a lifestyle change that includes dietary modifications, maybe weight loss, and exercise, need to be included in your new therapy.

If you take insulin as a type 2, your healthcare provider will teach you how to inject insulin, what type of insulin to buy, when, and how many units of insulin to take to bring down a high blood sugar reading. Or when to omit your insulin.

Then you start getting into a rhythm learning which types of foods don't shoot up your blood sugar, and you start to check more frequently because you want to keep your average blood sugar readings in the target range to delay or prevent diabetes complications.

You understand the importance of blood glucose testing and medical devices, medications and how they work. Feeling more confidant, you've got this down. Your healthcare provider is an integral part of your success now that you have an A1c target and made some dietary and fitness lifestyle changes. You are feeling unstoppable. You've got this. Knowing if you need to check your blood sugar more but are on a budget or limited by your health insurance, you can purchase lower-cost alternative glucose strips and meters, or apply for assistance from the medical device and medication companies.

Your Diabetes Has Been Demystified

Now that you understand how your medication works with the help of your healthcare professional team, you start tweaking it by watching what you eat and exercising, feeling successful because your blood sugars are becoming more consistent.

As a family member who has felt the deep pain of losing her mother, brother, aunt, and grandmothers to the disease, I want to help you figure out which part of the puzzle is missing for you. Once you get that last piece, you can have more confidence and validation from your A1c test, and experience how little changes may make a big difference in your overall health.

If you take away one thing from this book and implement it to achieve better blood sugars, it would make me happy. I would love to hear about your success, where you were stuck, and what helped you change. Email me at asknadia@diabeteshealth.com to share your story with me.

I care about your well-being. Even more important, your loved ones care more than you can imagine.

I want to share a few stories from my diabeteshealth.com online community. In particular, a type 1 and a type 2 story. Over the years, we have written up many inspiring stories about people living with diabetes who remind me that change is about having a certain mindset. It is not about willpower; it is about the desire to feel good mentally and physically.

Type 2 Success Story

Diabetes Health's Tanya Caylor interviewed Phillip Brenneman, a person with type 2 diabetes, who lost two hundred pounds without going on a diet and was able to get off his insulin and metformin.

How did Brenneman lose 200 pounds and get off insulin, metformin, and his cholesterol and blood pressure medications?

The Garrett, Ind., man says he did it one step at a time. Moreover, in the beginning, even that was more than he could manage.

Brenneman's first attempts at exercise took place in his chair at home. Arm circles and leg lifts were all he could handle when he decided, the morning after a Super Bowl party in 2015, that he had to make changes or risk missing his daughter grow up.

Sugar Happy

At 400 pounds, what people noticed was his weight. However, while that was the most visible part of his misery, he knew his type 2 diabetes was the real danger. He had watched his mother die from complications from that disease. Now in his mid-40s, he was on that same path and just a few years from the age at which she died.

Brenneman never went on a diet, per se. However, he did start reading labels and buying healthier food. Instead of picking up dinner at the drive-through, he began preparing veggies and lean grilled meats at home. The only processed foods in his diet were low-calorie products like Lean Cuisine frozen dinners and Skinny Cow treats. Eventually, he cut those out as well, preferring natural, organic fare he cooks himself.

After he lost 40 pounds or so, Brenneman joined the local YMCA. He started on the elliptical machine, eventually adding walking and jogging to his regimen. By the time he saw his doctor in October 2015, he had lost 120 pounds. His lab tests were normal. His doctor, stunned at the change, agreed to take him off his medications, provided he continues to monitor his blood sugar.

Brenneman eventually lost 200 pounds. His methods are not the quick fix people want to hear. He simply began to eliminate unhealthy behaviors and consistently worked to improve his diet and exercise habits along the way slowly. He now finds himself doing things that feel both comfortable and sustainable.

Having gotten used to the way premium foods fuel his body, treats that used to captivate him, no longer seem so alluring. For

Thanksgiving, he mashed cauliflower instead of potatoes. His family is on board with his lifestyle changes. His wife has lost 60 pounds and his daughter, now 5, is learning to love exercise. "We do not even plan on desserts," he says.

Brenneman, who has appeared on CNN and NBC's *Today* show, now says he checks his blood sugar more regularly than he did when he was overweight, generally at least once a day and whenever he feels "off."

"If I overload on carbs, I can feel it," he says. "It is never going to go away."

He has been able to control his blood sugar and maintain his weight loss by eating sensibly and exercising regularly. He completed his first half marathon in October 2016. The following month, he placed third in his age group in a 5K turkey trot. Though he is sometimes tired when his alarm goes off for his morning workout, he reminds himself, "that is just a mindset." He has learned that his body will respond once he begins working out.

"Most people know what they are doing wrong," he said. "You have got to own up to it. I am the one who put all that unhealthy stuff in my body." Now he is taking responsibility for his health, one step at a time.

Type 1 Success Story

Type 1 forensic scientist, Mark Ruefenacht, shares with me in an interview how he realized that dogs could be a major defense against life-threatening episodes of hypoglycemia. That insight led him to found Dogs for Diabetics ("D4D"), a Concord, California-based organization that trains dogs to alert their masters when they sense low blood sugar. D4D's website is located at www.dogs4diabetics.com/.

Nadia: How did you discover that dogs can sense low blood sugar?

Mark: In 1999, when I was on a business trip to New York City, a guide dog puppy, Benton, aroused me in the middle of the night from a low blood sugar incident, allowing me to get help. Whether Benton reacted to a change in scent or in the symptoms that I was exhibiting is unknown; however, that incident resulted in my idea of training a dog for this purpose.

Based on my background in forensic science, I am familiar with blood alcohol devices, which can differentiate alcohol-based problems from a low blood sugar event. I then spent several years studying dog scent training protocols for drugs, bombs, and search and rescue, as well as cancer detection. Along with extensive experimentation regarding the diabetic scent, I proved the capabilities of the dogs, and I developed a series of protocols that have been further tested over the last several years with well over 100 dogs. D4D currently supports over 80 client teams. Our longest working dog is Armstrong, with more than eight years of alerting experience.

Nadia: Does a dog have to feel a connection with a person to detect low blood sugar?

Obstacles That May Prevent You From Achieving Success

Mark: Many characteristics make a dog successful in a working relationship that provides this type of medical alert. One of them is the bond he develops with his companion. However, there are many other characteristics that both the dog and his handler initially need to become a consistent and reliable team. We have some criteria that we use to select the dogs for our training program. Our sources for dogs are primarily Guide Dogs for the Blind of San Rafael, California, and Canine Companions for Independence of Santa Rosa, California. The dogs they provide to our organization have been bred and trained from birth for service work.

With these excellent dogs and our proven selection criteria, we eventually place approximately 75 percent of the dogs that we train as members of working teams. That is a remarkable success rate when you consider the placement rate of other accredited service dog organizations. This is a good place to remind people that organizations that attempt to train pets or other non- service trained dogs will not meet the service characteristics for their dogs that comply with the requirements of the Americans with Disabilities Act for public access.

Additionally, while a small percentage of dogs will have a natural and strong drive to sustain this work ethic, most teams need ongoing support to sustain the process over the potential working life of the dog. Based on our experience, this has been a very clear issue.

Nadia: If you are in a public place and someone near you has a low blood sugar, will your dog alert that person, or is the dog trained to sense only your unique smell?

Sugar Happy

Mark: While the scent is universal, our dogs bond and work with their handlers. As such, they typically do not alert on others.

However, there have been incidents where this has happened. It can be a sensitive situation, given that not all diabetics are readily open about their disease, and some would prefer not to be identified. Accordingly, our clients are asked to be respectful as possible toward other people's privacy.

Nadia: How many scent sensory cells do dogs have?

Mark: The smelling receptacles for dogs vary by breed. The breeds of dogs that we train, Labrador retrievers and golden retrievers, have over 200 million sensory cells used for scent detection. Bloodhounds have over 300 million. Other breeds have fewer, but still can exceed 125 million scent sensory receptors. Dogs can discriminate scents at concentrations millions of times lower than humans, who have only five to 10 million scent sensory cells.

Nadia: How did you develop the science confirming that dogs can indeed be trained to smell low blood sugar?

Mark: I have extensive experience and training in scientific processes. The initial work that I did was to study existing information and work with professionals in dog scent training. There are many studies regarding scent training and the use of dogs in criminal work and other areas. The work that I did, pertaining directly to diabetes and low blood sugar, involved a significant experimental effort by myself and others in developing our protocols. It included type 1 people with diabetes and persons skilled in scent training for drugs, bomb detection, cadaver search, and cancer detection. We continue to have individuals in these areas consult for our program. We also have had the benefit of medical professionals who provide regular feedback, as well as scientific researchers who assist us in evaluating our processes and results.

Nadia: I have learned that some dogs give their owner a stuffed animal to alert the owner about low blood sugar. What's behind that?

Mark: I cannot comment on other programs' use of particular items to provide an alert. We have used a variety of techniques to have a dog indicate that it has detected the scent. Our preferred method is to use a bringsel, which is a small stuffed tube that hangs from the dog's collar or the client's belt loop. Our alert method was adapted from techniques used by cadaver search dogs. The dog is trained to hold the bringsel when it detects the scent. The objective is to have the dog provide the alert with a behavior that is distinctly different from normal dog behaviors, a sure sign as to what is occurring.

Nadia: If someone wanted to try training her dog to detect low blood sugar, could you give her instructions on how to go about it?

Mark: Training a dog to provide an alert to a potentially life-threatening condition is a serious matter. It requires a clear understanding of the medical condition, as well as dog behavior and training skills. Dogs have been known to assist their close human companions spontaneously, but the anecdotal information does not prove that it is due to scent recognition or empathy the dog may feel from the onset of serious symptoms. Scent training has the potential to provide an alert before the onset of the condition, while in these cases, the dog's recognition of symptoms is a reaction to the condition is present.

We believe that no one should undertake the training of dogs for this purpose without a clear understanding of all the risks. For an organization to attempt to teach untrained individuals to try to do this and then attempt to rely on a dog so trained is a recipe for disaster. Organizations attempting to provide training to individuals to self-train their dogs for this purpose do not seem to understand the full range of risks and will likely see a high degree of failure. Any program providing dogs for this purpose must have the appropriate background and quality assurance techniques and provide the ongoing support needed to sustain the working dog-handler relationship.

Accordingly, it is our policy to not offer advice on the training of dogs to detect hypoglycemia in nonprofessional trainers. There are medical risks that we cannot assume responsibility for without the ability to directly participate in or monitor both the dog and the diabetic's process.

Your Personal Take Away Notes To Remember

ACKNOWLEDGMENTS
AND THANK YOU

When I think back to 1990, when my former husband and I decided to start a mail-order diabetes supply store, I had no idea of the journey that would lie ahead of me. Diabetes was a word and lifestyle I was familiar with, but not in the way I came to live it. My former husband, who has type 1, is a model patient. My mother, who had type 2, illustrates all the habits one should *not* have to avoid diabetes complications.

Starting Sugar Happy Diabetes Supplies was an exciting venture for a new life. Having a mail-order business with no storefront, I was introduced to many people with diabetes while taking their phone orders. Calling in made my customers feel anonymous, which allowed them to feel free in sharing their most intimate diabetes stories.

As our home business outgrew our space, in six months, we found ourselves looking for a storefront. When I opened the storefront, it was exciting to finally meet some of these people because we already had a strong bond before meeting in person.

Over six years, I developed personal relationships with my diabetes customers. Our conversations became the inspiration for my next venture, *Diabetes on the Dial*, a live radio talk show that morphed from the conversations I had been having with my customers. Our discussions made me realize that there was much misinformation. It was clear to me that more people needed access to healthcare professionals who could give our listeners a second opinion on their diabetes self-management.

I would like to recognize two diabetes icons that have since passed; both were type 1s who contributed to my diabetes literacy — Kim Higgins, RN, CD, and Keith Campbell, RhP. Kim and Keith were both active in the American Association of Diabetes Educator. Kim passed away a few years ago, and Keith passed away this past year. Anyone who knew them will miss their genuine smiles and commitment to diabetes education and the community as a whole.

I want to thank the DiabetesHealth.Com print and online subscribers for their ongoing support. Without you, I would not be doing what I love to do. Thank you for all your support!

The lion's share of the *Diabetes Health* print magazines is a complimentary publication that is used as an educational resource in clinics, offices, hospitals, and support groups. Without my advertisers' commitment to my print and digital magazines, we all would miss these fantastic research reports and stories of our everyday heroes who inspire us to create change. With that being said, thank you, Trividia, Tandem Diabetes, Owen Mumford, Dexcom, UltiCare, BD, Asenscia, LifeScan, Inc., and Omnis Health. These device companies demonstrate their commitment to education by funding my efforts to serve you, the diabetes community.

A standout in her field, Laurie Jamieson's commitment to the McKesson Health Mart pharmacy patients, does not go unnoticed. Every year she orchestrates free diabetes magazines that serve the pharmacy community. If you are a Health Mart patient and receive *Diabetes Health* magazine, Laurie and her vendors are the people to thank.

My advisory board and healthcare professionals who have stood by our publications for almost thirty years are some of the most renowned healthcare professionals in their field. I would like to bring to your attention the most active voluntary board members: Robert J. Tanenberg, M.D., F.A.C.P. Professor of Medicine, Endocrinology, Dr. Richard K. Bernstein, John R. White, Jr., PA, PharmD Professor, Dept. of Pharmacotherapy, College of Pharmacy, Gary Arsham, MD Ph.D.; Jane Seley, DNP, MSN, MPH, GNP, CDE, BC-ADM, CDTC, FAADE, FAAN; Dr. Kathleen Palyo DNP BC-ADM; and Author Joy Pape, RN, Ph.D.

Their medical experience and some of their efforts in editing the chapters in this book, *Sugar Happy*, ensure that I meet the general diabetes standard guidelines.

Sugar Happy

Thank you, Patrick Totty, Monica Dennis and Katherine Schaaf for the time you have spent editing this book to ensure the best possible experience for my readers.

A special callout to my financial advisor Hal Jaffe, a hero in my life and a brilliant business counselor who has stood by my side as I continue to navigate through the changing publishing landscape.

My life would not be complete without the support of my children, Spencer and Miranda King; my brother John Edward Al-Samarrie; my sister, Mimi Al-Samarrie Bruce; and my good friends, Katherine & John Schaaf, Roxanne Araim, April Wolcott & Ted Wright, Lisa Baylacq, Greg Sison and Dr. Margit Süssman. These are all people who have stood by me emotionally and financially, cheering me on to my next endeavor.

Last but not least, my mother, Carol Louise McFeeley; my brother Jamal Abdul Malik Al-Samarrie; my aunt, Grace; my grandmothers Fatima and Helen and my former husband, Scott Millay King, continue to be teachers to me, in heaven and on Earth.

ABOUT THE AUTHOR

Nadia Al-Samarrie, Founder and Editor-in-Chief of *Diabetes Health*, received her Bachelor of Science from San Francisco State University.

Her *AskNadia* column is ranked #1 by Google and her DiabetesHealth.Com websites named "Best Diabetes Blog" for 2019 & 2017 by Healthline. With 24 nominations for her work, Nadia's efforts have made her stand out as a pioneer and leading patient advocate in the diabetes community. She produces and hosts a patient diabetes podcast in addition to her *Diabetes Health* TV interviews. She has been named one of the top 50 influencers in the diabetes space.

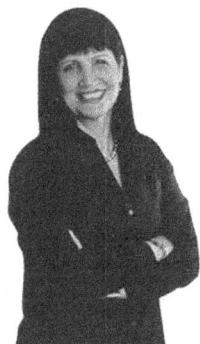

Nadia is also recognized as one of the longest most passionate, innovative diabetes patient advocates in the diabetes industry. Over 15 million copies of her magazine Diabetes Health is used in doctor's offices, emergency rooms, and pharmacies as an educational resource.

Sugar Happy

Under her reign- Diabetes Health magazine was named one of the top 10 magazines to follow in the world for 2018 by Feedspot Blog Reader.

Nadia was not only born into a family with type 2 diabetes but also married a type 1. She was propelled at a young age into "caretaker mode," and with her knowledge of the scarcity of resources, support, and understanding for people with diabetes, co-founded Sugar Happy Diabetes Supplies, *Diabetes on the Dial*, *Diabetes Interview*, now *Diabetes Health* magazine. She is best known for using her personal experience in writing articles on a variety of topics. Her mission is to investigate, inform, and inspire those living with diabetes.

Nadia has been featured on ABC, NBC, CBS, and other major cable networks. Her publications, medical supply business, and website have been sited, recognized, and published in Herb Caen, WSJ, Ann Landers, Lee Iacocca, *Entrepreneur* magazine, Brand Week, Drug Topics, and other media outlets.

Visit the website at diabeteshealth.com.

Contact Diabetes Health at press@diabeteshealth.com

Follow us on Twitter.com/DiabetesHealth

Contact AskNadia at asknadia@diabeteshealth.com.

THANK YOU

I hope my personal and professional commitment to you and my *Diabetes Health* family has demystified an important topic — your diabetes health. No longer feeling overwhelmed by what it takes to maintain good blood sugar levels in preventing complications, you are now ready to join my diabetes community, so I can continue to cheer you on and pick you up when diabetes burnout rears its ugly head.

As a Thank You for reading my book and demonstrating a commitment to your health, I would like to reward you with a free one-year digital subscription to *Diabetes Health* magazine, valued at $11.95. Simply go to diabeteshealth.com/free-magazine and sign up to receive your free magazine. You can skip the survey on the landing page by clicking "No Thanks," or you can answer the 14-multiple choice question. Your survey answers help me with my editorial direction. If I know what is important to you to read, then I can provide it.

Sugar Happy

Wishing you the best in health!

Nadia Al-Samarrie

Editor-in-Chief, *Diabetes Health*

AskNadia columnist and, most importantly, your diabetes advocate!

REFERENCES

Chapter 1

Diabetes Statistics. National Institute of Diabetes and Digestive and Kidney Diseases. https://www.niddk.nih.gov/health-information/health- statistics/diabetes-statistics. Sept. 2017.

Karvonen M, Viik-Kajander M, Moltchanova E, Libman I, LaPorte R, Tuomilehto J. *Incidence of childhood type 1 diabetes worldwide.* Diabetes Mondiale (DiaMond) Project Group. Diabetes Care. 2000 Oct;23(10):1516- 26.

Katsarou Anastasia, Claesson Rickard, Ignell Claes, Shaat Nael, Berntorp Kerstin. *Seasonal Pattern in the Diagnosis of Gestational Diabetes Mellitus in Southern Sweden.* J Diabetes Res. 2016; 2016: 8905474. Published online 2016 Dec 26. doi: 10.1155/2016/8905474.

Medications That May Increase Your Risk for Diabetes. National Research and Training Center, University of Illinois at

Sugar Happy

Chicago. http://www.cmhsrp.uic.edu/health/Diabetes_EDU/ Diabetes- 101/Medications_Increase_Diabetes_Risk.pdf.

Moltchanova EV, Schreier N, Lammi N, Karvonen M.

Seasonal variation of diagnosis of Type 1 diabetes mellitus in children worldwide. Diabet Med. 2009 Jul;26(7):673-8. doi: 10.1111/j.1464- 5491.2009.02743.x.

National Diabetes Statistics Report, 2017. National Center for Chronic Disease Prevention and Health Promotion. http://www. diabetes.org/assets/pdfs/basics/cdc-statistics-report-2017.pdf

*Diabetes Health Staff, Type 1.*5. Diabetes Health. https://www. diabeteshealth.com/type-1-5-diabetes/. Published January 6, 2009

Chapter 2

Central Pain Syndrome Information Page. National Institute of Neurological Disorders and Stroke. https://www.ninds.nih.gov/ disorders/all-disorders/central-pain-syndrome-information-page. May 25, 2017.

Smoking and Diabetes. Centers for Disease Control and Prevention. https://www.cdc.gov/tobacco/campaign/tips/diseases/ diabetes.html. April 23, 2018.

Weight Loss: Gain Control of Emotional Eating. Mayo Clinic. https://www.mayoclinic.org/healthy-lifestyle/weight-loss/in-depth/ weight- loss/art-20047342. Oct. 23, 2015.

Weisburger JH. *Eat to live, not live to eat.* Nutrition. 2000 Sep; 16(9):767-73.

Chapter 3

Campbell, Amy. *Diabetes Medicine: Alpha-Glucosidase Inhibitors.*

Diabetes Self-Management. https://www. diabetesselfmanagement.com/blog/diabetes-medicine-alpha-glucosidase- inhibitors/. Aug. 31, 2015.

Campbell, Amy. *Diabetes Medicine: Bile Acid Sequestrants and Dopamine Receptor Agonists.* Diabetes Self-Management. https://www.diabetesselfmanagement.com/blog/diabetes-medicine-bile- acid-sequestrants-and-dopamine-receptor-agonists/. Sept. 8, 2015.

Campbell, Amy. *Diabetes Medicine: DPP-4 Inhibitors.*

Diabetes Self-Management. https://www. diabetesselfmanagement. com/blog/diabetes-medicine-dpp-4-inhibitors/. Aug. 17, 2015.

Campbell, Amy. *Diabetes Medicine: Meglitinides.* Diabetes Self- Management. https://www.diabetesselfmanagement.com/ blog/ diabetes- medicine-meglitinides/. Aug. 3, 2015.

Campbell, Amy. *Diabetes Medicine: Metformin.* Diabetes

Self-Management. https://www.diabetesselfmanagement.com/ blog/ diabetes- medicine-metformin/. July 20, 2015.

Campbell, Amy. *Diabetes Medicine: Sulfonylureas.* Diabetes Self- Management. https://www.diabetesselfmanagement.com/ blog/ diabetes- medicine-sulfonylureas/. July 27, 2015.

Campbell, Amy. *Diabetes Medicine: Thiazolidinediones.*

Diabetes Self-Management. https://www. diabetesselfmanagement. com/blog/diabetes-medicine-thiazolidinediones/. Aug. 10, 2015.

Consensus Statement by The American Association of Clinical Endocrinologists and The American College of Endocrinology on

The Comprehensive Type 2 Diabetes Management Algorithm

– 2018 Executive Summary. American Association of Clinical Endocrinologists. https://www.aace.com/sites/all/files/diabetes-algorithm- executive-summary.pdf.

Consumer Guide 2018: Medications. American Diabetes Association. http://main.diabetes.org/dforg/pdfs/2018/2018-cg-medications.pdf.

Drugs, Herbs, and Supplements. Medline Plus. U.S. National Library of Medicine. https://medlineplus.gov/druginformation. html.

First Generation Sulfonylureas. National Institutes of Health. https://livertox.nih.gov/FirstGenerationSulfonylureas.htm. April 18, 2018.

Glycemic Targets: Standards of Medical Care in Diabetes—2018.

American Diabetes Association. Diabetes Care 2018 Jan; 41(Supplement 1): S55-S64. https://doi.org/10.2337/ dc18-S006.

Implications of the United Kingdom Prospective Diabetes Study. http://care.diabetesjournals.org/content/25/suppl_1/s28. American Diabetes Association. Diabetes Care 2002 Jan; 25(suppl 1): s28-s32. https://doi.org/10.2337/diacare.25.2007.S28.

Primary Prevention of Type 2 Diabetes. The Diabetes Educator. https://www.diabeteseducator.org/docs/default-source/legacy-docs/_resources/pdf/research/Primary_Prevention_Position_ Statement_TDE.pdf.

Toolkit for Implementing the Chronic Care Model in an Academic Environment: Oral Diabetes Medications Fact Sheet. Agency for Healthcare Research and Quality. https://www.ahrq. gov/professionals/education/curriculum-tools/chroniccaremodel/ chronic2a12c.html. October 2014.

Type 2 Medications. Diabetes Health. https://www. diabeteshealth.com/wp-content/uploads/2018/01/Type2.pdf.

Chapter 4

A Return to Normal, Pos-T-Vac Helps Me Over Come Erectile Dysfunction. Diabetes Health. https://www.diabeteshealth.

com/a-return-to-normal-pos-t-vac-helps-me-over-come-erectile- dysfunction/.

American Optometric Association's Annual Survey Reveals Misconceptions about Diagnosing Diabetes and its Related Eye Diseases. American Optometric Association. http://www.aoa.org/newsroom/aoa- annual-survey-reveals-misconceptions-about- diabetes?sso=y.

Aas Jørn A., Paster Bruce J., Stokes Lauren N., Olsen Ingar, Dewhirst Floyd E. *Defining the Normal Bacterial Flora of the Oral Cavity.* Journal List. J Clin Microbiol. v.43(11); 2005 Nov. PMC1287824.

Allahdadi Kyan J., Tostes Rita C.A., Clinton Webb R. *Female Sexual Dysfunction: Therapeutic Options and Experimental Challenges.* Cardiovasc Hematol Agents Med Chem. Author manuscript; available in PMC 2010 Dec 22.

Cardiovascular Disease and Diabetes. American Heart Association. http://www.heart.org/HEARTORG/Conditions/More/Diabetes/WhyDiabetesMatters/Cardiovascular-Disease-Diabetes_UCM_313865_Article.jsp#.WxIOX6kpA_U.

"Diabetes and Eyes, What Your Vision is Trying to Tell You." St. Louis Post-Dispatch. April 10, 2013.

Diabetes and Female Sexuality. Cleveland Clinic. https:// my.clevelandclinic.org/health/articles/7826-diabetes-and-female- sexuality.

Diabetes and Kidney Disease (Stages 1-4). National Kidney Foundation. https://www.kidney.org/atoz/content/Diabetes-and-Kidney-Disease-Stages1-4. November 2014.

Diabetes and Your Smile. Mouth Healthy. American Diabetes Association. https://www.mouthhealthy.org/en/az-topics/d/diabetes.

Diabetes Foot and Skin Care. National Diabetes Education Program.

Centers for Disease Control. https://www.cdc.gov/ diabetes/ diabetesatwork/pdfs/DiabetesFootandSkinCare.pdf. June 2017.

Diabetic Retinopathy. National Eye Institute. https://nei.nih.gov/eyedata/diabetic.

Diabulimia. NEDA. https://www.nationaleatingdisorders.org/diabulimia-5.

Female Sexual Dysfunction. Mayo Clinic. https://www.mayoclinic.org/diseases-conditions/female-sexual-dysfunction/diagnosis- treatment/drc-20372556. March 5, 2016.

History of Foot Ulcer Among Persons with Diabetes --- United States, 2000—2002. Centers for Disease Control. History of Foot Ulcer Among Persons with Diabetes --- United States, 2000—2002.

How to Lick Bad Breath and Dry Mouth. Live Science. https://www.livescience.com/5941-lick-bad-breath-dry-mouth.html. Dec. 23, 2009.

Knudsen, PharmD, CGP, Dawn. *How Medications Impact Libido.*

Pharmacy Times. https://www.pharmacytimes.com/ publications/issue/2010/june2010/lossoflibido-0610.

Menopause, Perimenopause, and Postmenopause. Cleveland Clinic. https://my.clevelandclinic.org/health/diseases/15224- menopause- perimenopause-and-postmenopause.

National Kidney Foundation. https://www.kidney.org/.

Trecroci, Daniel. *Erectile Dysfunction Common with Diabetes.*

Diabetes Health. https://www.diabeteshealth.com/erectile- dysfunction- common-with-diabetes/.

Ückert S, Oelke M, Waldkirch E, et al. Cyclic AMP and Cyclic GMP Phosphodiesterase Isoenzymes in the Human Vagina — Relation to NOS

Isoforms and VIP-Positive Nerves. https://www. medscape.org/ viewarticle/494280.

What Is Diabetic Neuropathy? National Institute of Diabetes and Digestive and Kidney Diseases. https://www.niddk.nih.gov/ health- information/diabetes/overview/preventing-problems/ nerve- damage-diabetic-.

Chapter 5

Checking Your Blood Glucose. American Diabetes Association. http://www.diabetes.org/living-with-diabetes/treatment-and-care/ blood- glucose-control/checking-your-blood-glucose.html. Feb. 7, 2018.

Clark, Stephanie. *Diabetes Health Type 2: Diabetes Diagnosis Creates More Stress for Women than Men.* Diabetes Health. https:// www.diabeteshealth.com/diabetes-health-in-the-news- product- diabetes- head2toe-plan/.

Gonzalez PHD Jeffrey S, Peyrot PHD Mark, McCarl MA Lauren A, Collins Erin Marie, Serpa Luis, Mimiaga, SCD, MPH, Matthew J., Safren, PHD. Steven A. *Depression and Diabetes Treatment Nonadherence: A Meta-Analysis.* Diabetes Care. 2008 Dec; 31(12): 2398–2403.

Sattley, Melissa. *History of Diabetes: From Raw Quinces and Gruel to Insulin.* Diabetes Health. https://www.diabeteshealth. com/?s=history+of+diabetes. March 3, 2016.

von Wartburg, Linda. *Type 1 & Type 2 Diabetes: Women and Sex.*

Diabetes Health. https://www.diabeteshealth.com/women-sex- and-diabetes/. Jan. 5, 2016.

Chapter 6

Clark, Stephanie. *Diabetes Health Type 2: Diabetes Diagnosis Creates More Stress for Women than Men.* Diabetes Health. https:// www.diabeteshealth.com/diabetes-health-in-the-news-product- diabetes- head2toe-plan/.

Checking Your Blood Glucose. American Diabetes Association. http://www.diabetes.org/living-with-diabetes/treatment-and-care/ blood- glucose-control/checking-your-blood-glucose.html. Feb. 7, 2018

Diabetes Sentry for Nocturnal Hypoglycemia. Diabetes Health. https://www.diabeteshealth.com/diabetes-sentry-for-nocturnal-hypoglycemia/. Sept. 16, 2015.

Family History of Diabetes Can Lead to Impaired Exercise Response. Diabetes Health. https://www.diabeteshealth.com/ diabetes-health-in-the- news-podcast-family-history-of-diabetes-can-lead-to-impaired-exercise- response/. Dec. 16, 2015.

More Exercise is Essential in Cutting Heart Failure Risk.

Diabetes Health. https://www.diabeteshealth.com/diabetes-health- in-the- news-podcast-more-exercise-is-essential-in-cutting-heart- failure-risk/. Dec. 30, 2015

Neugent, Brenda. *Short Walks May Work Best at Preventing Diabetes.* Diabetes Health. https://www.diabeteshealth.com/ short- walks-may-work- best-at-preventing-type-2/. May 15, 2018.

Thom, Sue. *Q&A: How to Lower Your Blood Sugar When It's Over 200 Mg/dl.* Diabetes Health. https://www.diabeteshealth. com/ qa-how-to-lower- your-blood-sugar-when-its-over-200-mgdl/.

Chapter 7

Connection Between Ketogenic Diet and Weight Loss Unclear.

Diabetes Health. https://www.diabeteshealth.com/connection-between- ketogenic-diet-and-weight-loss-unclear/. May 23, 2018.

References

Diabetes Exercise Essential in Cutting Heart Failure Risk.

Diabetes Health. https://www.diabeteshealth.com/diabetes-health- in-the- news-podcast-more-exercise-is-essential-in-cutting-heart- failure-risk/. Dec. 30, 2015.

Family History of Diabetes Can Lead to Impaired Exercise Response. Diabetes Health. https://www.diabeteshealth.com/diabetes-health-in-the- news-podcast-family-history-of-diabetes-can-lead-to-impaired-exercise- response/. Dec. 15, 2015.

Gold. Mari. Many Supplements Are Illegally Labeled. Diabetes Health. https://www.diabeteshealth.com/many-supplements-are- illegally-labeled/.

Diabetes Health. *High-Intensity Exercise, Not as Healthy as Believed.* Diabetes Health. https://www.diabeteshealth.com/high-intensity-exercise- not-healthy-believed/. July 14, 2017.

Neugent, Brenda. *Mediterranean Diet Again Linked to Lower Risk of Diabetes.* Diabetes Health. https://www.diabeteshealth.com/mediterranean- diet-again-linked-to-lower-risk-of-diabetes/. April 17, 2014

Neugent, Brenda. *Plant-based Diets Lead to Lower A1c Levels.*

Dietician of Canada Food Sources of Folate https://www.dietitians.ca/Downloads/Factsheets/Food-Sources-of-Folate.aspx June 2016

Diabetes Health. https://www.diabeteshealth.com/plant-based-diets-lead-to- lower-a1c-levels/. Dec. 22, 2014.

Preventing Exercise-Induced Hypoglycemia. Diabetes Health. https://www.diabeteshealth.com/diabetes-health-in-the-news-podcast- preventing-exercise-induced-hypoglycemia/. Dec. 9, 2015.

Stress Cancels Out Healthy Fat Benefits. Diabetes Health. https://www.diabeteshealth.com/diabetes-health-news-stress-cancels- healthy-fat-benefits/. April 6, 2017.

Study Examines How Exercise Can Affect Older Women Living with Diabetes. Diabetes Health. https://www.diabeteshealth. com/diabetes-health- in-the-news-podcast-study-examines-how- exercise-can-effect-older- women-living-with-diabetes/. Dec. 23, 2015.

Totty, Patrick. *The Hypoglycemia That Isn't There.* Diabetes Health. https://www.diabeteshealth.com/type-2-the-hypoglycemia- that-isnt-there/.

White, John. *Vitamins and Supplements: Taken for Health or Taken for A Ride?* Diabetes Health. https://www.diabeteshealth. com/vitamins-and-supplements-taken-for-health-or-taken-for-a- ride-2/.

Chapter 8

Alcoholic Drink-Equivalents of Select Beverages. Dietary Guidelines for Americans 2015-2020. https://health.gov/ dietaryguidelines/2015/guidelines/appendix-9/#table-a9-1- alcoholic-drink- equivalentsa-of-select-beverages.

Chapter 9

Free Diabetes Supplies and How to Apply for Them. Diabetes Health. https://www.diabeteshealth.com/ free-giveaways-4/.

The Cost of Diabetes. American Diabetes Association. http:// www.diabetes.org/advocacy/news-events/cost-of-diabetes.html. April 30, 2018.

Al-Samarrie, Nadia. *Type 1 Diabetes: Dogs That Sense Low Blood Sugar.* Diabetes Health. https://www.diabeteshealth. com/?s=dogs+for+diabetics. Nov. 26, 2015.

www.ingramcontent.com/pod-product-compliance
Lightning Source LLC
Chambersburg PA
CBHW032053090426
42744CB00005B/198